Me, Myself & My Amygdala
A Mindfulness Guide to Sobriety & Well-Being

BRIAN L. ACKERMAN, M.D.
Harvard Medical School Trained Psychiatrist

Illustrated by Jeff LeClair and Amara Merrit

What the Experts are Saying about this Book

"In his analysis of what may arguably be one of the most challenging issues for the human race to take on: both why we have impulses to self-harm and self-sabotage with alcohol and drugs, and what we can do about them, Dr. Ackerman offers his own fresh interpretation of mindfulness as a tool we can lean to utilize to be aware of these impulses, better understand than, develop a sense of mastery over them, and redirect them in the service of our self-care and well-being. His narrative takes the reader systematically through a process that includes a 'conscious shifting of attention' that can become as natural as regularly cleaning our 'mental windshields.' Infused with liberal use of metaphors, analogies, iconic references, and wonderful illustrations, *Me, Myself & My Amygdala* is a thoroughly enjoyable read in which Dr. Ackerman attaches a fresh and in-depth view of mindfulness with original ideas and concepts and a result that sticks. In our program, Dr. Ackerman runs a twice weekly mindfulness educational program for our patients which our patients eagerly look forward to because they are always learning something new about their brain, and therefore about themselves. For days after these groups our patients talk with their counselors, amongst themselves, and often with their families about the new concepts he introduces; like mental waste, mental basement, mental brake lining, mental dialysis and with his emphasis on learning, they learn to talk about and relate to their amygdala, the fight or flight area of the brain, in creative ways. They leave the group not only determined to maintain their goal of sobriety, but also to ensure that their amygdala no longer is running their lives. They feel less stigmatized by their 'addiction' and more understanding of their own humanity. Dr. Ackerman has also been a speaker at my class at Rhode Island College and to date is the only guest speaker mentioned and quoted in the class's final exam. In the final analysis, Dr. Ackerman demonstrates that he is a leading expert on mindfulness and its use in treating alcohol, substance use and mental illness and presents it in a way that is not only readable and enjoyable, but unforgettable."

—*Francis C. Spicola, Director of Intensive Outpatient Program; Community Care Alliance and Adjunct Professor of Psychology at Rhode Island College and formerly Executive Director of AdCare Rhode Island*

"Taking head-on the most challenging mental health problems on the era, Dr. Brian Ackerman, drawing on long clinical experience proposes an approach—to substance abuse and basic dissatisfaction—based on mindfulness and meditation. In this lively book, illustrated with technical drawings, cartoons, and explanatory diagrams, he provides a highly accessible format that incorporates novel formulations of psychology, neurology, and clinical examples galore. Professionals, patients and interested readers all stand to benefit from this exploration."

—*Thomas G Gutheil, M.D., Professor of Psychiatry, Harvard Medical School*

"Brian Ackerman, M.D. provides a refreshingly accessible approach to understanding and addressing addiction and the process of recovery. Through compelling, straightforward, clear thinking and innovative narrative Dr. Ackerman uses the framework of mindfulness training to give people with substance use problems a means to transcend negative thinking and achieve agency over their thinking and their behaviors.

"In *Me, Myself & My Amygdala: A Mindfulness Guide to Sobriety and Well-Being*, Dr. Ackerman gives patients powerful tools to counteract the harm they inflict on themselves with their addiction. It is difficult for patients and their treatment teams alike to reckon with how self-defeating behaviors result in chronic recurrent patterns of dis-ease. Dr. Ackerman has helped me, my staff and our patients grapple with the fundamental self-injurious drive built into the human brain. With this volume we not only learn how the neuroanatomy of the human brain impacts these behaviors but how through cultivating the brain's higher powers we can cultivate inner peace, well-being, self-caring and self-protection from the self-inflicted harm of addiction.

This book is a must read for all who suffer with alcohol or substance use, are affected by someone who does, or who is a treatment provider. It has inspired me to think differently; I think it will do the same for you.

—*Peter Kassis, M.D. FASAM, Regional Medical Director, Phoenix House of New England*

"Dr. Brian Ackerman's book on addictive behaviors posits that we can learn not just to change our minds but also change our brains, and thereby be effective in reducing our suffering. It's a path that relies on Mindfulness to help us better understand our instincts and enhance the role of the pre-frontal cortex as compared to the amygdala. At the basis of this work to transform our lives is caring for ourselves enough to seek change, something many of us were not taught but, encouragingly, can learn now."

Sharon Salzberg, author of Loving Kindness and Real Happiness.

"Finally, a book that respects individuals with substance use disorders as intelligent, curious, and compassionate human beings on a quest to better themselves despite adversity. Dr. Ackerman empowers and inspires people to better understand their own minds, actions, and motivations, so that they might in turn regain a sense of command and sense of self. I have seen this book in action and in person by watching Dr. Ackerman teach and practice: he gently guides people to better work with their own brains as competent, skilled navigators. This sense of purposeful action uplifts individuals from a place of helplessness and the resulting despair. Knowledge really is power and understanding the key to acceptance. When we learn about our brains, we just might, for the first time, truly learn about ourselves."

—*Katherine Anderson, LICSW, LCDP, QMHP. Former Director of Clinical Services, AdCare Rhode Island*

What Patients Who Have Used This Work Are Saying

"After 14 failed treatment efforts that focused mostly on 12 step approaches, I drove 14 hours to reach a treatment facility in Rhode Island where I sat in on Dr. Ackerman's presentation on substance use and the brain. Dr. Ackerman taught me that at the heart of addiction is the drive to self-harm, and that recovery depended upon walking away from victimhood and opening yourself up to a stronger, more powerful, more self- and other-caring, and self- and other-protecting self. These words were like a transformative wake-up call to me. I felt like I finally met someone who truly understood my disorder and truly understood me. Since then I have been able to rejoin my wife and children, stay sober, and we are busy planning a much more productive future. I stay in touch with Dr. Ackerman through Tele-Psychiatry. That his work is now available in book form is a blessing to all. Read this book, transform your life away from self-harm, and realize your healthy potential."

—*JBS*

"As a patient of Dr. Ackerman's for almost five years, I have reaped the enormous rewards of his mindfulness practice and psychoeducation on the topic a thousand times over. Mindfulness teaches you how to stop your brain in its tracks when base urges that drive harmful addictions and self-harming behaviors arise. As someone who struggles with serious self-injurious tendencies like cutting, entanglement in toxic relationships, and lots of self-sabotage, this has been life-saving and life-CHANGING for me. The book is like having access to Dr. Ackerman's therapy sessions 24/7—I can open up to the page I need and get the guidance I want without an appointment. The writing is intelligent, full of dry humor, and massively poignant, five out of five stars, I cannot recommend this enough."

—*Anonymous patient*

"As a successful businessman in my early fifties with a loving family and two young grandchildren, I didn't expect to find myself sitting across from Dr. Ackerman in a rehab facility for alcoholism. Having lost my battle with alcohol, I was contemplating a lonely and uncertain future. I was able to attend Dr. Ackerman's talk at my treatment facility days later about the connection between addiction and the brain, which was a real eye-opener for me. After discharge, I pursued doing individual therapy with him, got a proper diagnosis, and deepened my understanding of myself. He explained to me how alcohol was feeding the amygdala of my brain, causing it to be such a worthy opponent. Dr. Ackerman helped me realize that my battle was not just with alcohol, but also with my own brain and mind; a battle that was raging before alcohol even entered the picture. A year later, I am thriving, thanks in great part to Dr. Ackerman's guidance. I am thrilled that his guidance is now available to so many others in his new book. It's great! It's funny! It helps me remember all that I learned from him, and how learning to understand and overcome self-harming impulses is the key to keeping alcohol in the bottle, and out of my body where it just wreaks havok."

—*GS*

"Having practiced for 25 years as an Ivy league trained academic physician, I am well acquainted with the toll that stress exacts on ones' professional and personal life. In this, his first, book Dr. Ackerman distills the essence of his metaphor-rich techniques to deal with stress, e.g. "I choose not to board that train" (my wife and I call them 'Ackermanisms'). He masterfully integrates the anatomic, physiologic and psychological components of the brain to achieve emotional healing through their in-depth understanding. Read this book-you, yourself, and your amygdala will not be disappointed."

—LWD., M.D.

"As a member of Dr A's Mindfulness group for the past two years, I can say without hesitation that I have learned to distinguish my harmful and hurtful self-analysis from my enlightened and useful thinking. This has resulted in my making better choices in life while feeling much less anger and aggression. Dr. Ackerman infuses his writing with the same wit and humor as his weekly class, his fresh and down to earth approach, fully and clearly articulated in his book, helps others achieve self-understanding and acceptance. I give this book my highest 5 star rating and recommendation. I also give Dr. Ackerman my heartfelt gratitude for sharing his vision and extensive experience with the world."

—DH

"In these times when things feel their most chaotic, this easily readable and understandable book has the capacity to ground you and help you climb out of that tumult. It is engaging, has helpful tidbits for the moment, but most importantly to me, has a framework which can help you turn your amygdala on its ass …. or at least you can sit on it more comfortably. As a professional social worker and patient of Dr Ackerman, I find it an enormously helpful tool to which I refer again and again."

—JF

"I heartily recommend Dr. Ackerman's new book on mindfulness. I have been studying with Dr. Ackerman for several years. My life has been improved very substantially. I have learned to intercept negative emotions before they explode on my relationships. It is a process that takes awareness of the process, how to use it and practice. Importantly, I have learned to focus more time and energy on the activities that uplift and enlighten me. This has had very beneficial effects on my marriage and relationships at work, with my friends and others in my life. I have become more deliberate, thoughtful and much more positive, avoiding much more often the negative comments and instant reactions that can start a negative chain reaction.

"*Me, Myself & My Amygdala* explains this well in an easy to read narrative using many effective analogies. Whether or not you suffer from substance abuse (I do not), this book can be a breakthrough in your life, no matter how you are doing. No one is perfect. This may well bring you to a higher level of satisfaction with your life."

—RF

Me, Myself & My Amygdala:
A Mindfulness Guide to Sobriety & Well-Being

Copyright © 2020 Brian L. Ackerman, M.D.

Produced and printed by Stillwater River Publications. All rights reserved. Written and produced in the United States of America. This book may not be reproduced or sold in any form without the expressed, written permission of the author and publisher.

Visit our website at
www.StillwaterPress.com
for more information.

First Stillwater River Publications Edition

Library of Congress Control Number: 2020919790

ISBN: 978-1-952521-49-2

1 2 3 4 5 6 7 8 9 10
Written by Brian L. Ackerman, M.D.
Illustrated by Amara Merritt and Jeff LeClair
Published by Stillwater River Publications,
Pawtucket, RI, USA.

TEXT SET IN MINION

Publisher's Cataloging-In-Publication Data
(Prepared by The Donohue Group, Inc.)

Names: Ackerman, Brian L., author. | Merrit, Amara, illustrator. | LeClair, Jeff, illustrator.
Title: Me, myself & my amygdala : a mindfulness guide to sobriety & well-being / Brian L. Ackerman, M.D., Harvard Medical School trained psychiatrist ; illustrated by Amara Merrit and Jeff LeClair.
Other Titles: Me, myself and my amygdala
Description: First Stillwater River Publications edition. | Pawtucket, RI, USA : Stillwater River Publications, [2020]
Identifiers: ISBN 9781952521492
Subjects: LCSH: Substance abuse--Patients--Rehabilitation--Popular works. | Recovering addicts--Mental health--Popular works. | Mindfulness (Psychology) | Well-being. | Self-control.
Classification: LCC RC564.29 .A35 2020 | DDC 616.86/03--dc23

The views and opinions expressed in this book are solely those of the author and do not necessarily reflect the views and opinions of the publisher.

Personal Dedication

To my father Arnold Ackerman, who, at times was contentious growing up, but who role-modeled many invaluable traits. He was a chemist. Working in his lab as a kid sparked my interest in science. He was an avid stamp collector and a life-long student of religious study. While I was neither interested in stamp collecting or religious study, from his stamp collecting, I learned to observe and pay close attention to those details which truly distinguish and make something especially valuable. From his lifetime of religious study, I learned to devote a lifetime of study, which for me is to help improve our understanding of our-selves and of human nature.

After, my mother died late in life, he also became more than a father; but a true friend, a real-life reinforcement of one of the important themes of this book: the patient pursuit of our best selves. As humans we are all works in progress, as are our relationships. He was also keenly interested in education. I know he would take great pride in this book.

Dad, this book is devoted to you.

Professional Dedication

To my three mentors, my 3 kings: Osho, George Gurdjieff, and Charles Darwin whose clarity of thought reflected in their writings and lifetime devotion provided me sumptuous meals of food for thought—which I digested, recombined, seasoned with 40 years of psychiatric clinical experience, and reformulated in these writings. Osho could take a subject matter like the difference between loneliness and aloneness and speak intelligently about the difference for hours. Gurdjieff rigorously applied the tool of self-observation, which in my work becomes observing both our higher and lower self. Darwin applied the tool of careful observation of the natural world, to generate ideas which upon reflection became formulations (Higher Level, Meta-Thinking), which in turn became the Theory of Evolution and of Natural Selection, ideas so compelling and useful that they need not fear extinction. If Darwin's work was the careful observation of the natural world, mindfulness is the careful, compassionate observation of our internal mental life. It is my sincere hope that the meta-level ideas I introduce here; like **mental waste** and **mental dialysis** will be both serve as a testimony to the trees that others have planted generations before me, as well as bear mental fruit for generations to come.

    I would also like to dedicate this book to the scores of neuroscientists like Michael Gazzangia and Antontio Dimasio, Richard Davidson, primatologists like Frans De Waal, and the pioneering ever emergent Mindful-ologists like Dan Siegal, M.D., Jon Kabot-Zinn, M.D., and Jeffrey Schwartz, M.D., who have been trail-blazers in bringing mindfulness-based approaches to mainstream healthcare.

    I would also like to give two resounding shout-outs. One is to Steven Pinker, who serves for me as an alive and current role model helping all of us through his genius, knowledge, clarity of thought, study of language, and writings, to learn how to better think about, and integrate science, neuroscience, evolution, history perspective taking, intelligence, reason language and wisdom, so that we can better direct our psychic energies both outwardly and inwardly to our better angels, to help us realize and enhance our problem-solving capabilities and our well-being.

My other shoutout is to author and poet Mark Nepo. With the delicate brush strokes of his writing, Mark helps us more fully realize the soul in nature, as well as the rather unique soul of our human nature that is perhaps too keenly aware of its own imperfections.

And finally, I dedicate this book to both the hundreds of thousands of alcohol and substance suffers who share their heart-breaking stories day in and day out, calling out to us all, as if they are on a tube adrift a sea for HELP, as well as the countless partners, ex-partners, parents, children, siblings, step-family members, friends, neighbors, counselors, nurses, doctors and administrators who tirelessly swim out to try to rescue them. **Alcohol and substance use are life threatening and debilitating disorders**.

This book, like a hurricane chaser, is designed to help us all get up close and personal with **our human brain which comes factory-equipped with a suitcase full of tumult even before a substance or drop of alcohol is added to the combustible mix we are born with**. As we learn to see more clearly the built-in maelstrom of our dueling nature, we can begin to more intelligently chart a path to a true and lasting recovery.

Consider me your personal guide as I am about to take you on a tour of your brain and your two minds. (Did you know you had two?) Like a good snorkeling instructor, I will try to help you appreciate your rather amazing brain. On a snorkeling tour you get to see beautiful fish and coral, as well as learn to beware the barracuda and sharp coral.

On my brain tour will get to see your magnificent prefrontal cortex and learn to avoid stepping on the sharp amygdala. If I accomplish my mission you will discover that what you see is fascinating and when you get back on the boat to catch your breath you will be looking forward to the next opportunity to look again and see what else you can see about yourself and others.

Are you ready to dive in?

Table of Contents

Foreword .... *xiii*
Acknowledgments .... *xv*

1. What is Addiction? 1
2. How it Starts 3
3. What is Mindfulness? 8
4. Understanding the AMYGDALA 12
5. The Evolutionary Perspective 15
6. Mental Digestion 32
7. The Purpose-Driven Mindfulness 43
8. Excremation Points 53
9. Negative Thinking 57
10. Meta-Thinking 62
11. The Evolution of the Human Minds(s) 67
12. The Role of Trauma 77
13. Role of Medication 79
14. Understanding the Prefrontal Cortex 83
15. Mental Waste 94
16. Cravings 96
17. Mental Dialysis 99
18. Duel Diagnosis 108
19. Schnapps-is 116

Appendix *120*
Teaching Metaphors in Me, Myself & My Amygdala *124*
About the Author *129*

Foreword

I became a psychiatrist because I found the brain to be the most interesting organ in the body. I have yet to meet a human being who is not interested in the brain. The brain is an organ of survival. We are the only living entity that is aware we have a brain, have the capacity to study it, and learn how to optimize its incredible capabilities. However, there are many thoughts, feelings, and impulses produced in this same organ of survival that lead us to self-hate and self-injure, and to behave in ways that actually threaten and undermine our very survival. Yes, our human brain, the best brain on the evolutionary market, contains an impulsive, self-harming component to it, but its most unique feature is its capacity to be aware of its own self-harming impulses and ability to learn to correct for them. To understand self-harm, we need to not only look microscopically at the at our brain's neurotransmitters, but also step back and see the big picture of ourselves as human beings how we evolved and how we are still evolving.

In this book, I propose that **alcohol and substance use disorders are really self-injury disorders** and address the two fundamental questions connected to self-injury:

1. **Why do humans self-injure?**
2. **How do we learn to manage more effectively our self-injurious impulses?**

I also propose that we can learn how to understand ourselves so much better to the extent that we understand how our human brain works. In the spirit of the new decade, my hope is this book helps us all take a step closer to learning how to **see ourselves with 2020 vision.**

My undertaking is ambitious for sure. But given the explosion of new information about the brain even in the last 20 years, I am hoping to at least synthesize information from many related fields. This book asks us to consider that if we were to Google

BRIAN L. ACKERMAN, M.D.

an owner's and operator's manual for our brain that included care instructions, what might it say? At the very least, I hope that upon reading and digesting what I have written, YOU will be able to operate and care for your brain more effectively, to live a healthier and more peaceful drug-free life, and to help others you love and work with (or have tried or are trying to love and live with) to use and care for their brains more constructively as well.

—Brian L. Ackerman, M.D.
July 3, 2020

Acknowledgments

My work has been supported by so many staff, administrators, co-workers, and patients, friends and family.

David Lauterbach was the former CEO of the Kent Center who hired me in 2016 and supported my vision of incorporating mindfulness therapy groups and staff training into the center, and I want to thank his successor Daniel Kubas Meyer, who kept the flame burning brightly. Dr. Lillya Koyfman, medical director there who enthusiastically refers all her anxious patients to my mindfulness group.

Peter Mumma, CEO of Phoenix House NE is a visionary who recruited me to be Psychiatric Medical Director and incorporated these groups into the weekly treatment of all in-patients.

Fred Trepazzi, AdCare CEO, who sponsored mindfulness staff training as well as weekly patient groups. He didn't just direct staff to come to the presentations—he came himself.

Dr. Kazi Salahuddin, medical director, of the Community Care Alliance who, as one of his very first activities as the new medical director, sat in on one of my mindfulness therapy groups to see what all the buzz was about. I also will thank Richard Crino, who is an unstoppable force creating innovative mental health outreach programs. Special shout outs go to Frank Spicola and Kim Griffith at CCA. My very first mindfulness therapy group for alcohol and substance use was launched in Woonsocket, and over the past four years, this modality of treatment has spread to Providence, Warwick, North Kingston, and Exeter, Rhode Island.

Special thanks to the illustrator Amara Merrit, a RISD student who embraced and infused this book with her artistic, creative eye, hand, and spirit. Also to Myra, who painted the last picture "Baggage You Don't Need to Carry," and of donations, like from my daughter Avra's butterfly garden—the fabulous vegetable garden in JF and BF's backyard. Those pictures are there to remind us all that it is so much better to grow a lush garden than to be a lush!

Lastly to Jeff LeClair, who came through with some last-minute graphic design heroics. Pictures can help us see and understand so much better.

A special, special shout out to my wife LuAnn, who helped me navigate what I still consider the Twilight Zone of word documents, formatting, the internet, JPEGs and are they the X-files?

Special thanks to my mentors and highly esteemed psychiatrists: Drs. Thomas Gutheil and George Vaillant for their draft-reading and cogent editorial input.

Special thanks and gratitude to all those who took the time and made the effort to read the book draft and who provided input and feedback: Daneisha, Kate, MB, JS, GS, DL, JF, BF, WL, Kate Anderson, Frank Spicola, Dr. Peter Kassis.

Finally, to all staff, students, and patients who have worked hard to incorporate this work into their lives and work, as most exemplified by the homework examples included in the book, and the Woonsocket group member who every time he runs into me in the parking lot, shouts out from his car: "Hey Doc, honk if you're aware of your amygdala!"

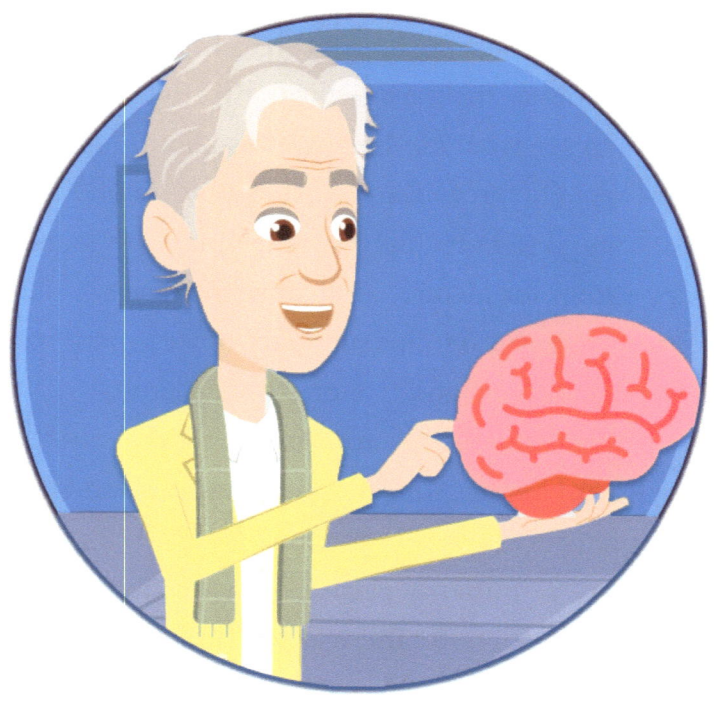

What is Addiction?

Addiction is the repeated use of alcohol or substances despite the rather horrific and known long-term negative consequences.

While there are many variables that drive this disorder, the main ones that mindfulness directly addresses are the self-injurious, self-harming, self-neglecting, and self-hating thoughts and feelings which are derived from the lower psyche and propel the substance use and self-injurious behavior.

The mindfulness definition of an addiction is a SELF-INJURIOUS IMPULSE DISORDER.

The mindfulness-based treatment teaches us that we can become AWARE of these self-injurious impulses and learn that they are coming from a really small part of our brain: our AMYGDALA, which is smaller in size than an acorn. We can learn that it is this part of the brain that presses us to self-injure and disregard the consequences. While the amygdala is inside us; it does not truly represent us. We also learn to be AWARE that it is our much larger, grapefruit sized, PREFRONTAL CORTEX, which is the home of our self-caring and self-protective impulses. Our prefrontal cortex is our true representative and the home of authentic "I". The mission of MINDFULNESS is to help us learn how to get our PREFRONTAL CORTEX to become LARGE AND IN CHARGE!

This book asks to wonder: **How can we operate our brain optimally?** What is required for its care? Whether I buy a car, a lawn mower, or a washing machine, they all come with operation and care manuals. I need to know what buttons to push to get whatever I am using to work properly, as well as what buttons not to push. I need to know what to put in it; as well as what not to put in it. Some buttons like cruise control on a car I may never use. The "button" that mindfulness training teaches us to push to get our brains to operate optimally is our prefrontal cortex.

This is our mental G-spot: the brain area we need to access and develop to find true satisfaction, contentment, and inner peace. Also, if you read the brain's care instructions it will say quite clearly: The brain consists of live cells and tissues. Do not put anything toxic into your body that will reach your brain! **Your brain requires a healthy, pollutant-free environment to operate properly**. Alcohol and substance use are toxic to all the cells in the human body and are particularly toxic to our brain cells.

Given that our brain is the vital organ of our survival, we can begin to see that we are effectively shooting ourselves in the foot, and self-sabotaging by putting anything into our bodies that could harm or interfere with its optimal functioning. **In order for us to function optimally, we need our brain to function optimally.**

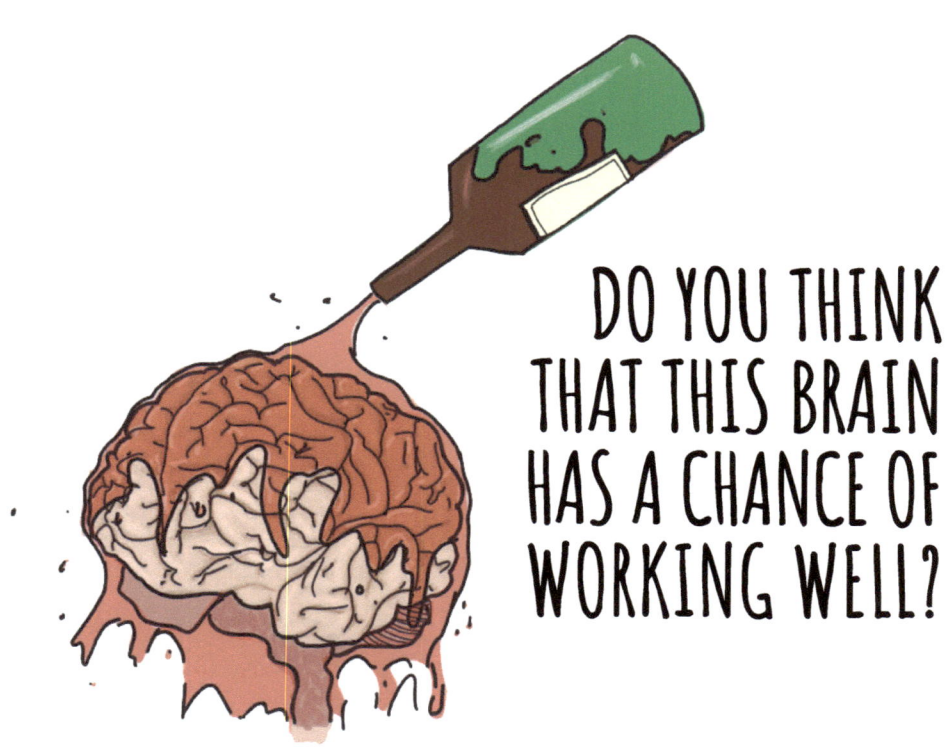

How it Starts

Most people start using alcohol and drugs for fun, socializing, and to take the edge off of their moodiness, anxiety, or the stresses of their daily lives. Most believe that they can stop their use anytime, and really don't see themselves as venturing into the precarious world of self-medicating. At first, they are—or at least act—clueless as to what they are really getting themselves into, whether that be smoking their first cigarette or smoking crack cocaine.

However, it does not take long before one cigarette becomes a pack-a-day habit, and the fentanyl use requires using Narcan to keep oneself alive.

Central to this disorder are the obsessive preoccupations with getting the drug, romanticizing and glorifying its benefits, and compulsively using it despite the distress and often dire consequences that accompany it.

Recently, I hired a contractor recommended to me by someone I trusted who had done a lot of work in our home. After a few weeks on the job, the contractor reported he needed $1000 for more material, which I wrote a check for. He took the check and never returned to the job. We soon learned that later that week he had been arrested and sent to jail for the armed robbery of a convenience store apparently to get the money to buy more crack cocaine. When I learned of this, I recalled a brief conversation with him 2 weeks earlier when he learned of my expertise in treating alcohol and substance use disorders and indicated that he wanted to talk to me at some point about a 'friend' of his who had significant drug use issues but who refused to get help.

Unfortunately, this story is not at all atypical of the extremes that users will go to get their fix. He had a great job but gave it all up for a drug fix and ended up with a felony rather than the satisfaction of a job well done. I also learned the true meaning of the phrase to 'pay through the nose!' The stories of self-sabotage abound and are rather dumbfounding.

The urge to get a hit often becomes so compelling that some start leaving work in the middle of the day. Parents will stop meeting their parental obligations or even use while their children are left unattended. Once use starts in earnest, the moral compass seems to go out the window. I know of drug users who readily steal money from their family members to buy their drugs, and others who without hesitation, will steal their family member's opiate medicine prescribed for their cancer treatment. Dishonesty and deceit become the norm as if this is just what you have to do to make it as a user.

In an experimental study of rats in 2009, it was learned that rats given the options to self-administer cocaine and or self-administer food and water, only self-administered the drug and actually then died from starvation and dehydration as a result. The initial pleasure sensation caused by the infusion of the drug, acts as a powerful reward and reinforces the self-administering behavior. Rats have no capacity to realize that it is their lower circuits that press them to self-administer.

Humans, however, have a prefrontal cortex: the brain module which allows us both conscious awareness and our capacity to learn about our brain's lower neuronal circuits and hence our drug vulnerability. This lower circuit awareness can help us realize the often misguided and life-threatening nature of these lower circuits, and problem-solve how to over-ride them.

From this perspective, addictions—whether they involve gambling, sex, or substances—can be seen as disorders of misdirected motivation. It is not easy to swallow the horse pill: the notion that we share these lower circuits with animals.

However, it is more comforting to learn that we have other neural circuits which they don't, located in our prefrontal cortex, which provides us with a Get Out of Jail Free card. Unfortunately, learning how to use this card often requires expensive learning and lots of practice. The out-of-control-drug seeking, the lies, deceits and associated crimes will leave a user with rather intense feelings of isolation and rejection, which likely contributed to the drug usage in the first place.

Treatment centers exist to help users detoxify safely from their use, as well as try to interrupt this vicious cycle of alienation seeking relief through drugs, which leads to more alienation, which in turn is followed by even more drug-seeking. Mindfulness training adds another dimension, which is inviting the user to get interested in learning enough about their brain so that they can begin to envision how they can learn to employ their best neural circuits.

NEGATIVE THOUGHT SPIRAL

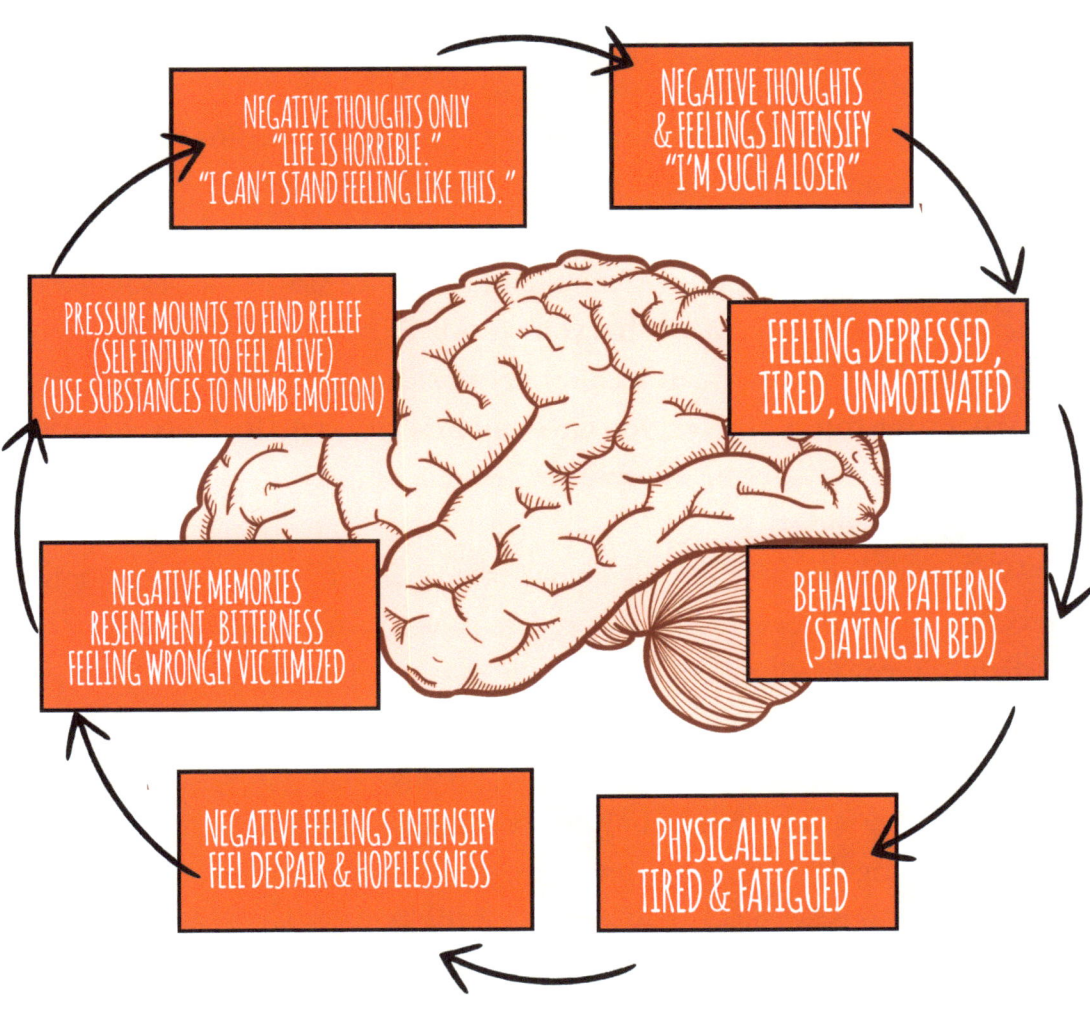

What they learn about their lower neural circuits is they are part of the brain's powerful primitive reward system designed to motivate us to eat and drink sufficiently as well as mate. Often users are aware of a more general lack of motivation they feel in life, and then use drugs to try to jump start their motivation, only to find out that the only thing they become more motivated to do, is use.

This effectively converts their 'survival instincts' into a death march. From this perspective, addictions, whether they involve gambling, sex or substances, can be seen as **disorders of misdirected motivation.**

Alcohol and drug withdrawal can be life-threatening, causing seizures, and resulting in brain and body damage.

Overdoses are life-threatening. Alcohol and drug usage also increase suicidality, which is life-threatening. Alcohol and substance use are far more serious than simply having a few too many that you quickly recover from the next day.

When you repeatedly put alcohol or substances into your body without true regard for the consequences, you have embarked on a path of self and other injury that will have devastating adverse consequences for you, your body, and anyone you truly care about.

When you learn how to utilize your brain correctly, you will stop going in this direction, get your bearings, check the map, and resume your journey to your true destination: your well-being.

Getting lost does not have to be a life sentence.

For most, the 'high' of the first use is the best. Users then begin a chase to recreate that first 'fabulous' experience only to learn that tolerance develops quickly, and that even increasing doses doesn't come close to generating the initial high.

Tolerance simply means that over time the same dose produces a lesser effect. This is often why most drug users are multi-drug users and so often combine many substances or switch their so-called drug of choice often in a 'vein' search for their secret sauce.

Addiction results from the effect of repeated drug use especially on the amygdala area of the brain. Of great importance here is that the worst brain changes and harm occurs in this one area and much less so in the rest of our brain. Visual, hearing, motor, and balancing parts of the brain remain largely undamaged.

Our prefrontal cortex is also largely spared so that while they may have quite a snowstorm in their driveway, a crucial initial goal of a mindfulness-based approach is to help users realize they still have very good and underutilized parts of their brain real estate; their snowplow to help make a path to get out, and that there are people there who will help them learn how to better utilize it.

Once a brain area is sensitized to a substance, it just does not feel right without it. Without the drug present, the changed brain starts a form of protest—better known as withdrawal—that is experienced throughout the body. The particular symptoms of which vary with which drug has been used and in what amounts.

Most drugs only last in our systems only a short while. Cocaine leaves the system in just 1 ½ hours, which then coils the spring for the repeated use to keep the fix going—the driver of the addiction. Another line, another drink, is needed to keep the current buzz going and more is needed in the morning to avoid the discomfort of withdrawal. It's a sinkhole.

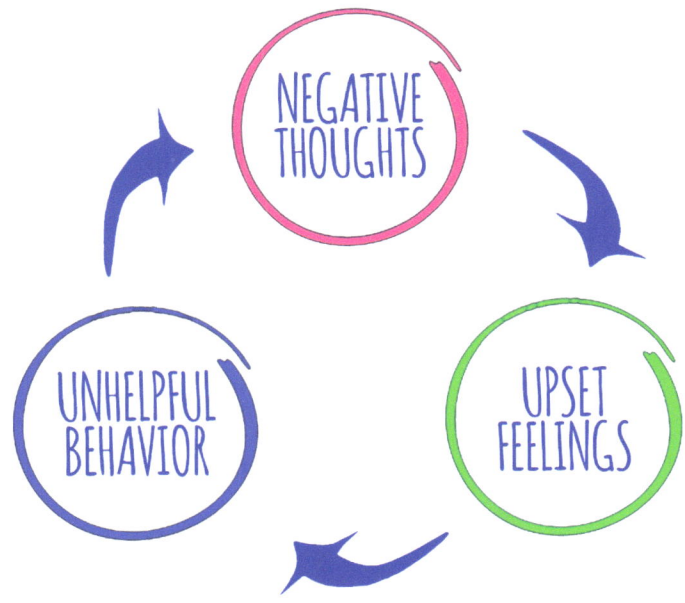

What is Mindfulness?

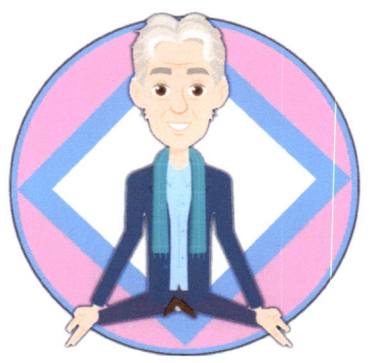

Mindfulness is training ourselves to become compassionate witnesses to our internal mental life. It entails learning about the brain and learning that our sense of ourselves is derived from only two very different portions of our cortical real estate. We effectively live in a mental duplex with our best and higher self living upstairs in the prefrontal cortex, while our worst or lower self occupies the downstairs apartment.

Our best self literally sits on top of our worst self. As we learn to look at ourselves holistically, we can see that even our very sense of ourselves is but a small mental portion of our brain's broad functioning, and that there is a lot more going on in our brain than our mental components. We learn in mindfulness that we are not our brain, and that our brain serves many more functions than providing a home for our best and worst selves.

Mindfulness teaches us how to distinguish those thoughts, feelings, impulses, attitudes and behaviors that are derived from our higher versus lower self. It then teaches us to shift our attention so that we guide ourselves to actually refocus our attention to the best area of our brain and mental functioning (the home of our well-being and inner peace), and away from the fight or flight area of our brain and mental functioning (the home of our fear, anxiety, anger, aggression and thoughts of being defective and deficient).

Mindfulness helps us to cultivate the awareness that we have not one but two selves, and these selves are in constant conflict. Mindfulness is the ever-evolving awareness of our double nature. It also teaches us how unwittingly we have become identified with our worst self, and have presumed that what comes from the fight or flight area is our true self—whereas this part, is but a small, hardwired primitive part of our brain.

What is Mindfulness?

This brain module—**our amygdala—is a thorn in our side, and in the side of ALL human beings.** We learn this thorn—our hard-wired, built-in IED: Improvised Explosive Device, needs to be identified, handled with care, and disarmed if we are to stop hurting ourselves and hurting others, and get on with living.

Me, Myself and My Amygdala, teaches us that we are not only not our brain, but most definitely, we are not our amygdala. Mindfulness teaches us to become a compassionate witness to, but not identify with, the amygdala.

It also teaches us that it is the prefrontal cortex is the area of our brain which is the most evolved, and affords us the unique mental function of inner mental awareness that enables us with a specialized form of double vision. The prefrontal cortex is aware of (can see) itself, and at the same time is aware of (can see) all the other brain regions including the amygdala which is often in direct conflict with it.

Mindfulness teaches us that the prefrontal cortex is the region of our brain which is the home of our capacity for love, compassion, inner peace, joy, and well-being. The really good news is that the best part of our brain is huge, and this part has tripled in size from our predecessors.

Finally, and most importantly, the prefrontal cortex is open through neuroplasticity for development and strengthening.

Neuroplasticity is the brain's capacity to generate new neurons and new connections amongst those neurons through *practice and learning* to *become even more fabulous*. We know now that we can do **more than just change our minds; we can actually change our brains**. The positive impact of practicing meditation and mindfulness on the brain can be seen on brain scans.

The prefrontal cortex is the part of our brain we need to learn to identify with. This is the fertile part of the brain in which we want to grow our tomatoes (so to speak), and from this part we can have a genuine sense of "I". It consists of collections of neuron networks that function like teams, which through practice and learning become even more fabulous at what they do.

The point of the title: *Me, Myself & My Amygdala* is to help us all transition from where we all start: overidentifying with our amygdala and what oozes out of it. To be

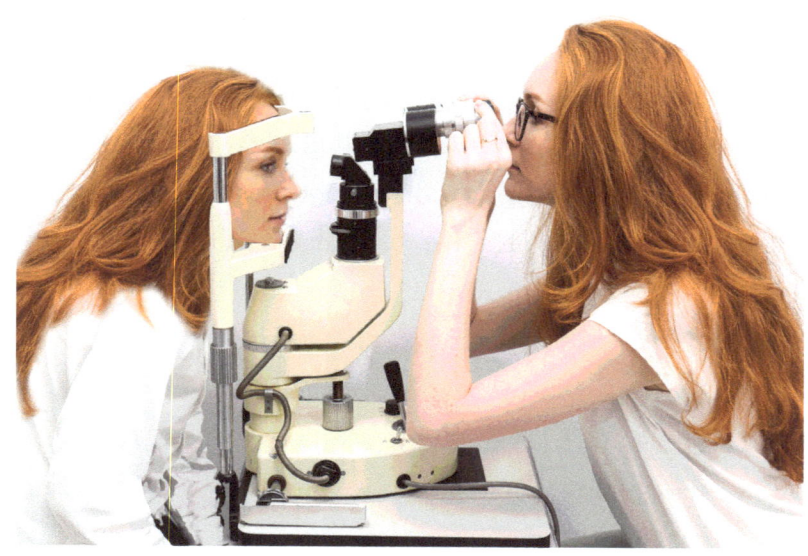

truly able to **see ourselves with 2020 vision**, we will need to transition and learn to see our new and evolving selves as: Me, Myself & my prefrontal cortex**.** Mindfulness practice helps us to increase and strengthen the connections in our prefrontal cortex.

Our prefrontal cortex allows us to be aware of our lower psychology. ALL human beings have a lower psychology, just as all human beings have a temper. We can learn to pro-actively keep this lower psychology from dominating our lives. Our best self

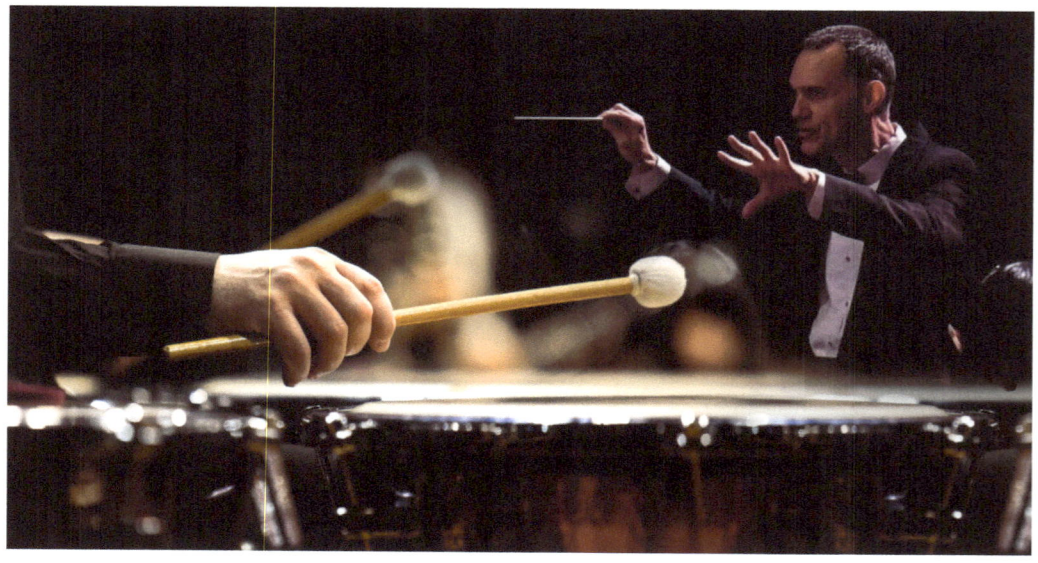

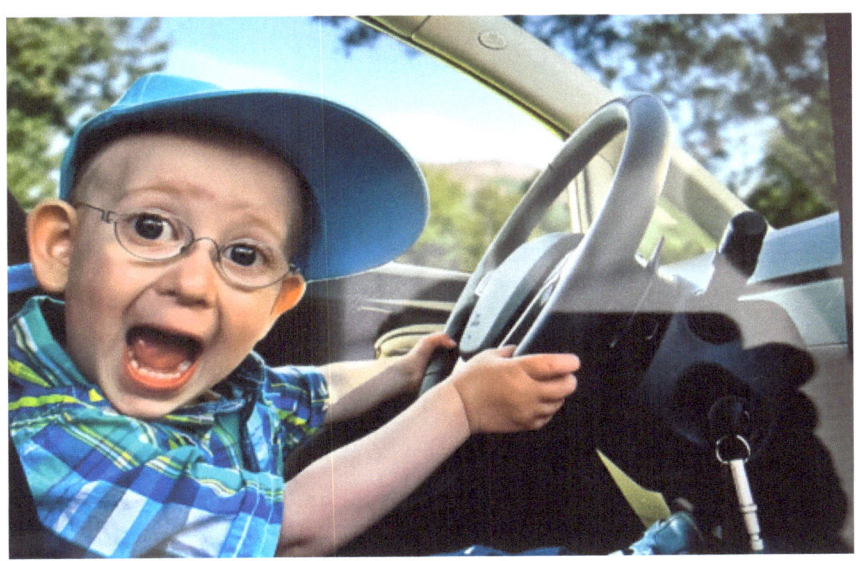

is not only fabulous, in and of itself, but because it is open for development and is also is the home of our aspirations (who we are striving to become). It represents our upside potential. All human beings are works in progress; we are evolving. Our prefrontal cortex is so unique that it allows us to reflect on our thoughts, feelings, attitudes, impulses, and behaviors. Beyond this reflection, this meta-thinking, it also the gives us the capacity to modify each and every one of these.

The human brain is an amazing organ, especially if we learn to harness the various brain modules to work more effectively as a team. Our brain modules are like the various instruments in an orchestra. The prefrontal cortex is like the conductor whose mission it is to bring out harmony of the whole from the various contributing instruments. The conductor understands that the amygdala is like the drum which when played thoughtfully, adds emphasis and punctuation; and if not, just makes noise.

The thesis of this book is that **if you are suffering mentally and with the use of drugs or alcohol**, **your little amygdala is running your life**; which makes as much sense as giving your three-year old the keys to your car.

The keys to your recovery lie in getting your prefrontal cortex to take the keys back and putting the three-year old part of your brain in the back seat of the car, with the seat belt on carefully fastened.

Understanding the AMYGDALA

The amygdala is a small primitive part of the brain also known as the fight or flight area. In all mammals that preceded humans, the amygdala occupied a larger percentage of the brain, especially relative to the size of their prefrontal cortex (which in humans, is quite large). The amygdala functions like an alarm system to pick up signs of danger, and activates neural circuits in its possessor to fight the danger or to run like hell. This is the brain module where fear and aggression are produced. Pre-human, the aggression from the amygdala is directed outwardly to a predator or a potential food source.

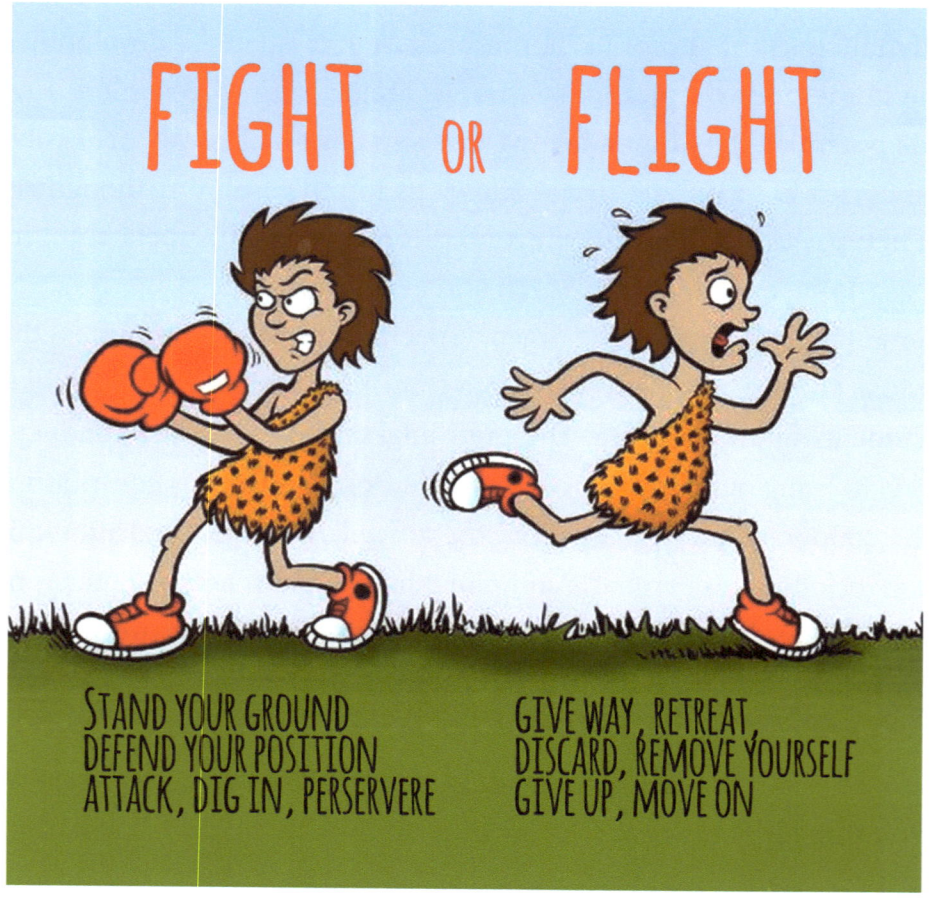

Understanding the Amygdala

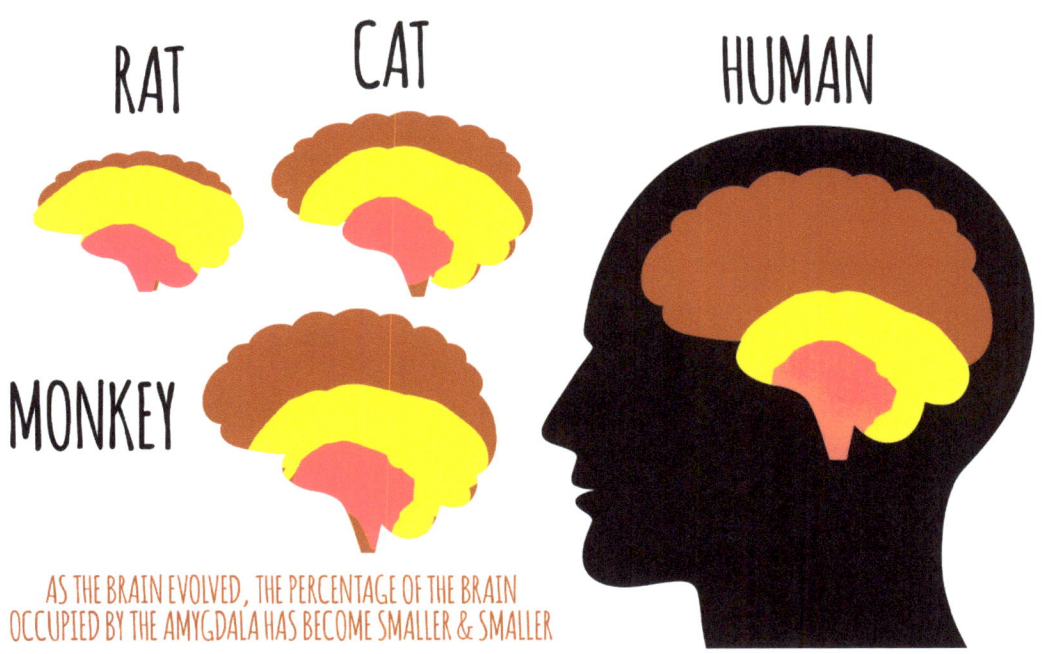

AS THE BRAIN EVOLVED, THE PERCENTAGE OF THE BRAIN OCCUPIED BY THE AMYGDALA HAS BECOME SMALLER & SMALLER

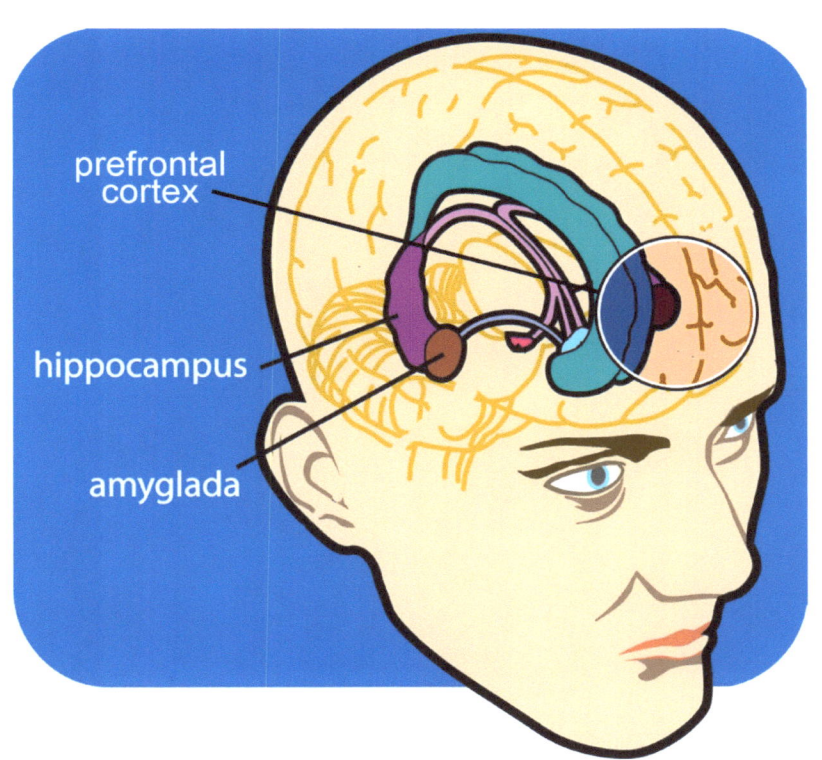

As the brain evolved, the percentage of the brain occupied by the amygdala has become smaller & smaller

In human beings, our aggression is bi-directional—and is not only directed outwardly, but inwardly as well. Unless your name is Mike Tyson, you are not likely to bite others, but are more likely to make biting comments *about* others. However, as human beings, we direct the greatest percentage of our aggression toward ourselves.

We are the only living entity who recognizes ourselves in the mirror, but if we pay attention to our inner commentary when we see ourselves in the mirror, it is all negative. We simply and automatically don't like what we see, and in the blink of an eye we are saying "ugh" to and about ourselves.

It is to this automatic thought stream that mindfulness directs our attention. It is essential that we become aware of this and interrupt and change this negative "mental reflex".

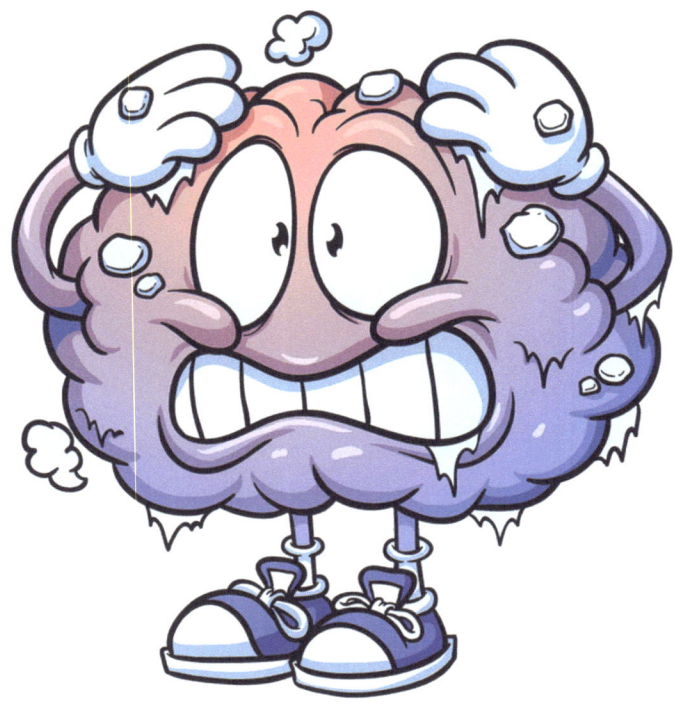

The Evolutionary Perspective

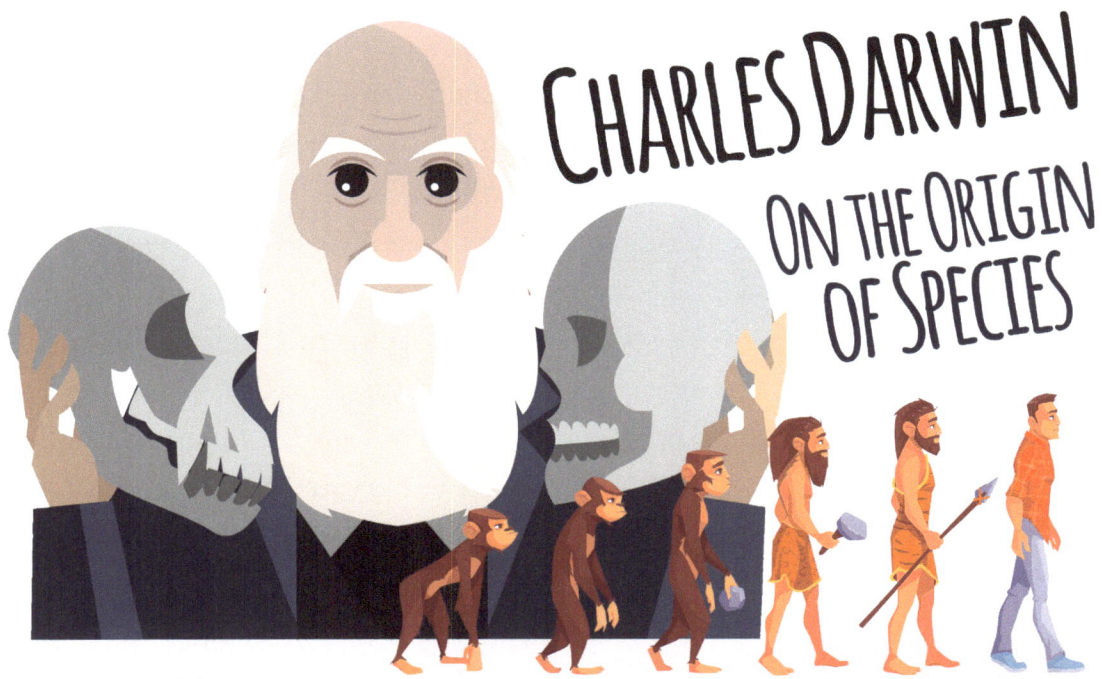

Evolution has taught us that human life exists on a continuum with other living organisms, and that even the physiology of the cell-building block of the brain—the neuron—is essentially the same in a squid, as it is in humans. Beyond that, we share ninety-eight percent of our genes with apes, and a staggering high percentage with other primates. While we are similar to the species from which we evolved, by definition, we are also quite different. **It is not the strength of our bones and muscles that makes us unique; it is our brain** and in particular, the way our brain is different from that of our predecessors.

Our brain is not the largest; a whale's brain is 5 times larger. Many small animals have large brains relative to their size and weight. Our brain is 3 times the size of that of a chimp, with the largest increase made to the prefrontal cortex. Perhaps as many as 50 billion species have lived. 500 million years ago there is evidence of the very first brains, while it was only 200,000 years ago that the first human brain arrived on the scene.

Body cells, in some ways, are like leaves on a tree. They grow, fall off and are replaced. Our bodies contain 37 trillion cells. Every day 60 billion are replaced. The human brain has 100 billion cells. Every day 86 million of them are replaced.

While the degree of brain cell replacement is unique to humans, the basic nerve cell itself is not. The basic elements of nerve transmission exist as far back as single celled organisms as different chemicals inside the cells and different ion gradients. Those of which, inside versus outside the cell, generated Western Union-like Morse coded electrochemical signals and transmissions.

Our brains and neuron circuits were formed to allow our behavior to become more organized, efficient, and effective. Some of the very first brains that evolved in fish were located behind the eyes, and provided signals for them to find food, mates and dodge predators. Not all living things have nervous systems, but a nervous system evolved like our phone systems to more efficiently send and receive information from a distance.

A nerve allows a living organism to interact with its environment by transducing the information it receives from its receptor neurons to its response generating neurons, effectively allowing a stimulus from the environment to generate a response.

We can think of a brain as a sensory motor integration device. This simplest stimulus-motor response is a reflex as represented by that of a bi-valve that enables the mollusk to sense danger, close its shell, and withdraw. The sensation of danger is received by one part of the clam's elementary sensory nerve.

Then the signal is transduced, and another signal is sent along an elementary motor nerve to a ligament to contract and close the shell. In a behavioral metaphor, the doorbell rings (the stimulus); then we open go to the door and open it (the motor response).

Human behavior still has many reflexes such as the eye blink—which like the clam, quickly closes the eyelid to help protect the vulnerable and essential eye from danger. We also have the knee jerk reflex, which while it involves sensory and motor nerves, does not even involve our brain, as the reflex arc only goes only through the spinal cord.

Mindfulness training proposes that some of our behavioral responses from the lower part of our brain are more akin to spinal, automatic reflexes than true higher cortex evolved responses. This explains why some of our thoughts and some of our behavior are more automatic and are done without a true higher thinking quality to it. We need to aware of, identify, and learn not to get hijacked by lower automatic, thoughts, feelings and impulses. As life evolved, and higher-level transductions became beneficial, stimulus signals were sent to a higher-level central headquarters for processing and assessment, which led to the development of the first more centralized brain.

Some species like octopus are considered to have a separate brain in each one of their eight legs. Evolution then moved in the direction of centralizing separate brains under one roof, in a way that resembled what happened when separate stores began to open together in a mall. It seems we have many smaller brains within in our bigger brain, organized within a hierarchy.

Our brain's in-built organization is rather remarkable, but like a teenager's room or a government, it is capable of even better organization yet.

One of the unique features of the human brain is its capacity to change and reorganize itself and in effect evolve itself; whereas with preceding brains, the circuits you were dealt genetically largely determined the hand you could play. We typically don't like the temper card we are born with, but with mental skill learning and training we learn to 'snowplow' the rising upset and inhibit the release to try to avoid hurting ourselves or others.

Mindfulness teaches us that we are capable of a sufficient measure of brain reorganization, and that we can learn to more effectively optimize our brains.

Teaching ourselves how to do this, like learning a musical instrument, shooting a 3-point shot, or cooking a fabulous recipe is one of the ways **our brain is unique and not restricted to its original wiring and programming**.

We know that the increased myelination of the brain up to age 30 helps our brain to function more efficiently and effectively. This biological process may be what is required for a teenager to finally pick up the mess in their room and put their clothes away. However, we are also able to mature psychologically, as well as biologically—and this psychological maturation requires education, evolved perspective taking, and learning to become more selective in managing our competing thoughts,

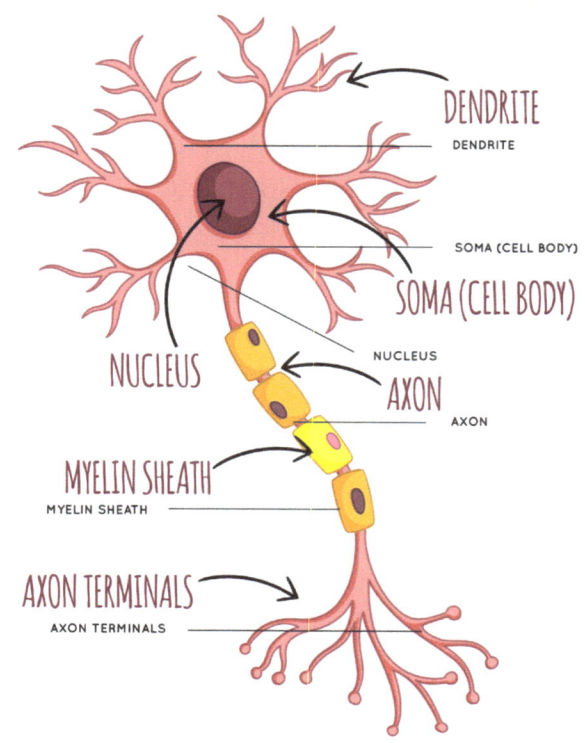

feelings and impulses, so that we can make wiser choices in how we act. We learn that **we can rewire and reorganize the best part of our brain with effort and training.** Our goal is to help ensure that the best part of our brain is in our driver's seat, paying careful attention to the road, resisting the impulses from another part of our brain that pushes us to look elsewhere and take our eyes off the road.

The centralized brain and the nervous system developed to organize, coordinate, and execute many essential functions under one roof. It evolved to execute functions that could not effectively be governed by simple reflexes, where lots of sensory information needed to be gathered, collated, and considered in relationship to past memories and future anticipations, to be processed more reflectively than reflexively acted on. We can understand the urgency of developing systems that could detect and respond to predators, as well as access food sustenance and water. These systems evolved like a government or a business.

Over time, many departments were formed that needed to be organized and coordinated. Like a company rapidly expanding, as the brain's business began to boom, we can imagine how the first 100 neuron "employees" of the company were given more specific roles as the company expanded. The waiting room receptionist neuron developed the skill set to run the food-shopping department, while the bookkeeper neuron became the foreman of glucose and oxygen regulation. The sales manager became the regional manager for sensory information, sight, smell, sound, taste and touch. Another ambitious set of neurons were placed in charge of motor movements. Areas of the brain—like schools—were opened as designated learning areas for remembering, reasoning, and problem-solving.

The most senior, capable, and creative future-thinking neurons—the ones who seemed to more fully understand the company's core business of staying alive and thriving—were assigned to the executive office suite and put in charge of oversight of the company's success and future. An integral part of their job was to align activity with the company's mission to stay alive and thrive. Toward that end, it also needed to be able to make proper assessments of the competition, handle all potential threats and enemies, anticipate and prepare for shortages, and creatively adapt products for an unknown future, which would continually unfold.

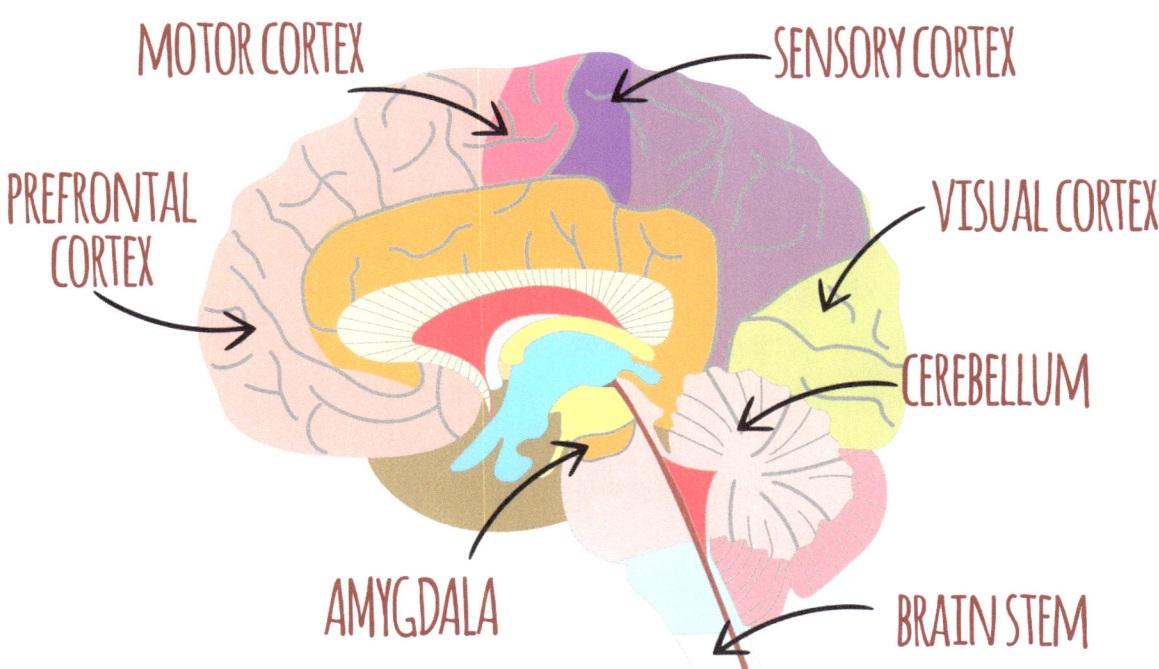

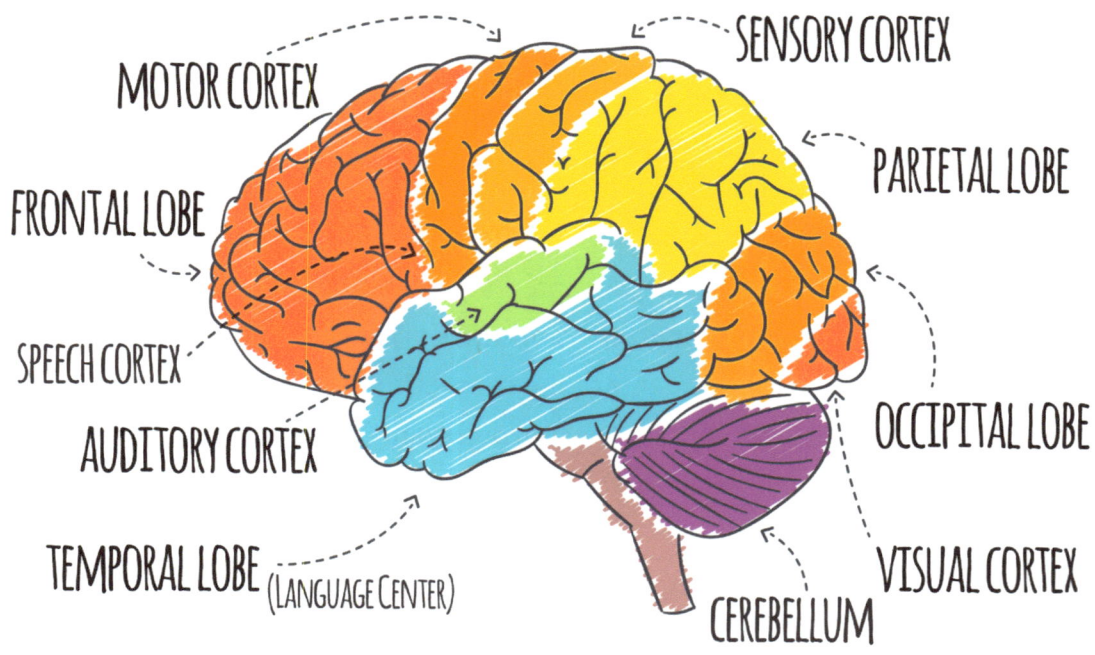

While humans have one centralized brain, it is at times helpful *to* **think of our one brain as consisting of many sub-brains housed under one roof**. While each of our sub-brains has a vital function, each sub-brain is not created equal in its utility or mode of action. The parts of our brain lying closer to the spinal cord tend to generate more automatic, quicker and reflexive responses; while the parts closer to the top of our brain are more reflective and considered. While slower, they handle more data and generate more complex and nuanced responses.

The lower-level departments process the incoming signals, handle what they can, and pass the higher level information along either to highlight it, or cross it out. By the time it gets to the CEO's desk located in the prefrontal cortex, the great quantity of information is whittled down to help enable a more considered, yet still relatively quick, response.

We know that neurons develop specificity of functions, so visual neurons become specialists in translating the information provided to the visual cortex. They start off like medical students all in the process of becoming physicians, but as they develop, become specialists in various areas of medicine. Some become surgeons or dermatologists, while others remain primary care physicians. Even within the visual cortex, there is further sub-specialization, as some neurons are geared to detecting size and shape, others to color, and others yet to whether or not what is being seen is moving, how fast, and in what direction.

The brain area that has expanded most in humans over our mammal and primate relatives is our prefrontal cortex. Our prefrontal cortex is twice the size of our nearest primate relative.

This expansion of our cortex gives humans beings higher level cognitive capacities which enable us to: understand and comprehend abstract concepts, reason more intelligently, speak and understand language, imagine and rehearse things in our mind before doing them, be creative and flexible, think outside the box, take different perspectives—and perhaps most importantly—select what we pay the most attention to.

Our prefrontal cortex allows us to have a sense of 'self'—and the even more abstract concept of competing selves—to have and understand abstract thoughts to generate hypotheses, understand symbols and language, appreciate the sense of the passage of time, create and play music, to be aware of on inner-self talk, to mentally rehearse before acting or deciding, to problem-solve, and to plan ahead. This neuronal grouping in our prefrontal cortex also gives us our rather unique quality of inner awareness that allows us to be aware—unlike any prior form of life—that we have a brain and an inner mental life. Our remarkably increased cognitive capacity helps us realize just how much we underutilize this capacity. Mindfulness training teaches us to be aware of this underutilization and correct for it.

Our inner mental life is really quite strange. One of the essential functions of mindfulness training is to help us step back from our inner mental life and learn to become a compassionate witness to it. **Becoming a compassionate witness to oneself is central to meditation and mindfulness training.** Many years ago, I had the good fortune to go on a safari in Kenya, which allowed me the opportunity to watch the rather amazing wildlife come to watering holes while we travelers watched with awe and amazement, silently and safely from close by, perched in high cabins overlooking the watering holes. I did not realize at the time that this **silent, awe-inspiring, witness centered in curiosity** would become central to my meditation training many years later.

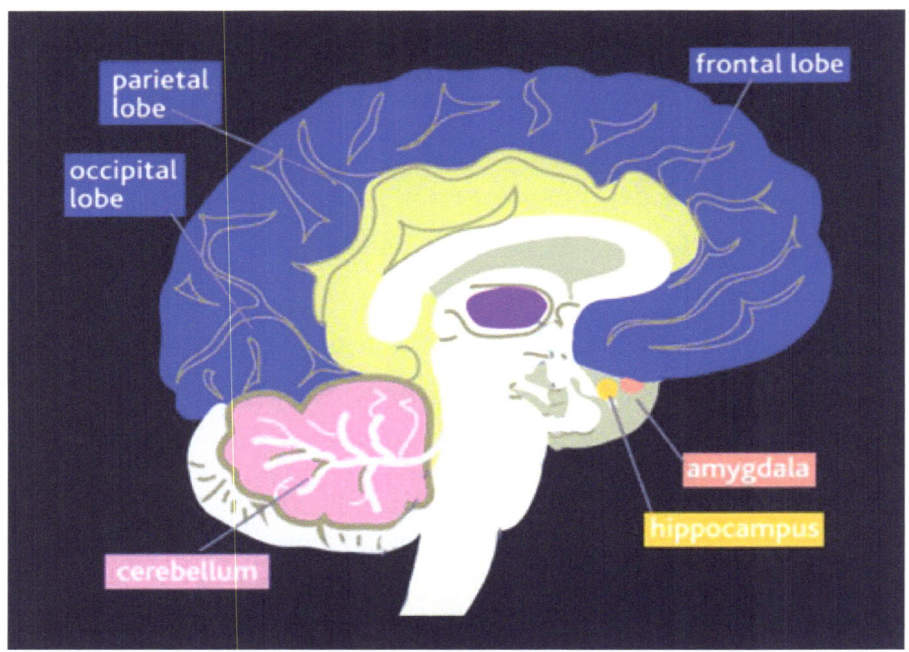

The difference was that instead of witnessing a live aardvark and its rather unusual elongated nose at a watering hole, my meditation training taught me how to become a compassionate witness to the aardvark-ness of the human mind. Mindfulness training invites us to become as curious about our inner mental life as we might become about the rather amazing wildlife. It calls upon us to be become non-judgmental witnesses to our wild and woolly thoughts and feelings. It calls on us to develop and train this rather unique capacity to become a witness. We might say that a giraffe is unique because of its long neck, and surmise that the purpose of this unique feature was to allow it to access food at the tops of trees where there was less competition. We can see the giraffe's long neck is a unique feature that has survival value.

Mindfulness training teaches us that **our inner awareness is a unique feature of humans that in turn has survival value.** When we witness just how often we come across swampy areas of thoughts and feelings, we must learn to remember that there are larger spring-fed mental watering holes just around the corner from the swamp, so that we don't drink the first water we come to no matter how thirsty we may be.

Because we are aware that we have a heart, we have the survival advantage of being

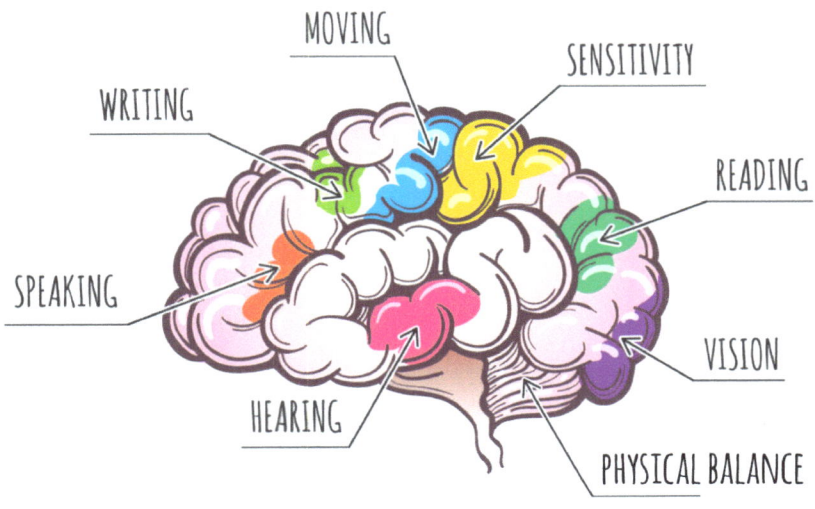

able to study the heart and learn about it. We learn that it is a vital pump made of muscle that can be strengthened. We also have the survival advantage that we can understand the abstract concepts—such as the purpose of the heart to deliver oxygenated blood and retrieve carbon dioxide-laden blood for lung excretion. We can understand the concept of basic hydraulics, and how our vital pump might become stressed if the vessels it pumps blood through have become clogged in any way. We can also understand and utilize the abstract concept of cardiovascular fitness, to motivate us to exercise more and strengthen our pump's muscle, quit smoking (or at least smoke less), and eat better to reduce the clogging, and understand just how important it is to direct a portion of our life energy and time to build our cardiovascular fitness.

Pause for a moment to **consider just how many survival advantages we receive by possessing this unique capacity for inner awareness in our brain,** and for a unique quality of learning that allows us to study, brainstorm, and apply what we can learn to our survival advantage. Mindfulness training helps us not only to appreciate this capacity, but also to cultivate it, develop it, and apply it wherever it can be beneficial. Because we realize how crucial our visual acuity is to our survival and well-being,

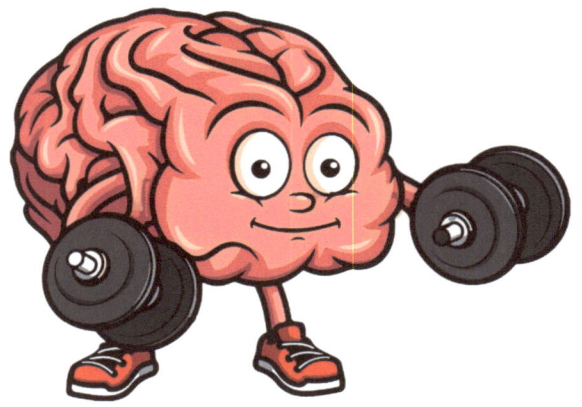

we take the necessary steps to get glasses and contacts to correct and optimize our vision. Mindfulness training helps us all realize just how impaired the way we see ourselves is. Mindfulness training is the necessary step we take to **learn how to see ourselves with 20-20 vision!**

Because we understand that our heart is such a vital organ, we become immediately more motivated to take better care of it. With this understanding in mind, Mindfulness training then directs us to apply the same principals to the awareness of our brain as yet another vital organ. Like the awareness of having a heart, the awareness of having a brain allows us to study and learn about the brain. If there is cardiovascular fitness, surely there must be **brain fitness** and **mental fitness.**

Mindfulness training teaches us that there are parts of our brain that work just fine as they are, and other parts that we can strengthen and better optimize in a way analogous to physical fitness training. It also teaches us how to recognize and learn how to free ourselves from all that clogs our mental arteries. Fortunately, evolution has provided us with **Neuroplasticity—our neurons ability to replace themselves and form newer and stronger connections with other neurons as a direct means to improve our brain and our mental fitness**.

The ability of our neurons to make new connections is the essence of all new learning. **The Laws of Neuroplasticity demonstrate that the frequently used areas of the brain expand, while underutilized parts shrink and atrophy.** Armed with this knowledge, mindfulness training directs us to **actively and purposely strengthen our prefrontal cortex, while also actively and deliberately work to shrink our amygdala**.

How do we do this? To strengthen the prefrontal cortex, we intentionally practice doing more of what the prefrontal cortex does: we reflect more, we meta-think more, we problem-solve more, we learn more, we practice catch with our positive thoughts feelings and impulses more, and we become more aware of and amused by (but not hijacked by) the oozings of the amygdala. A good friend of mine lived his life with what I consider a very useful adage: "Learn something new every day!"

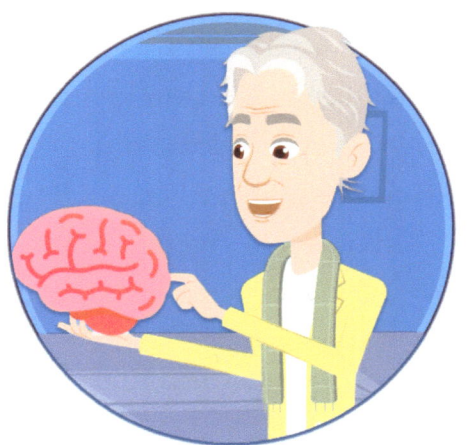

What we learn matters less than the fact that we are learning. The proviso is that what we are learning is truly beneficial to us.

Whether we are learning to change the tire on our car, cook a new recipe, or learning a new song, new language, or a musical instrument, our prefrontal cortex is engaged, active and being strengthened. In similar fashion we want to become aware of and intercede in anything that might strengthen the amygdala area. Anger, anxiety, bitterness, resentment, negative self-thinking are all amygdala activities, and the more of our psychic energies we spend with these thoughts and feelings, the more the very area we are now trying to shrink actually expands. Mindfulness training directs us to be aware of and empowered to direct and re-direct our psychic energies accordingly.

This is a 3-step process: 1) awareness of what is on our 'mind', 2) determination as to whether it is useful or non-useful, followed then by 3) the shifting of attention off of what is non-useful and onto what is useful and beneficial.

Since we now realize **how essential it is to our well-being to shrink our amygdala,** we have another even more compelling reason to not use drugs or alcohol, think negative thoughts feelings or impulses, or waste our psychic energies craving for drugs. All these things simply strengthen the very area of the brain which, if left unchecked, is the nemesis of every human life.

Mindfulness training teaches us to become compassionate observers and witnesses to our inner mental life, to become amused by how odd it is, and especially to learn not to identify with most of its oddball content. Freud's great discovery focused on the strangeness of our unconscious dream life. But mindfulness training helps us learn to pay even more attention to our conscious thoughts, feelings, and impulses.

When we do this, we realize just how odd and influential our conscious mental life is. Freud connected our mental suffering to our unconscious mental lives, which then needed to be revealed in order to find relief; whereas mindfulness training teaches us that our conscious mental life is fully capable of creating and sustaining our mental anguish.

This is not to say that there are not also important unconscious issues as well that may need to be uncovered and addressed. One central focus in mindfulness is cultivating the awareness of the push and pull we experience alternately in the direction of self-harm or self-care. There are often many unconscious issues buried in them darn hills.

Those who have been subjected to abject mental abuse, neglect, or physical and sexual violence, or have been given drugs to use as kids by their own parents, may be oblivious to having picked up in their own conduct where their parents left off. Now it is they who have become the abuser, and their body and their sense of self has become the abused.

Another dynamic is the "I'll cut off my nose to spite your face" syndrome, where effectively substance use becomes a statement like: "If you didn't take care of me properly and protect me from harm, how do you expect me to protect myself?"

There is an angry, embedded message in their conduct, which says in effect:

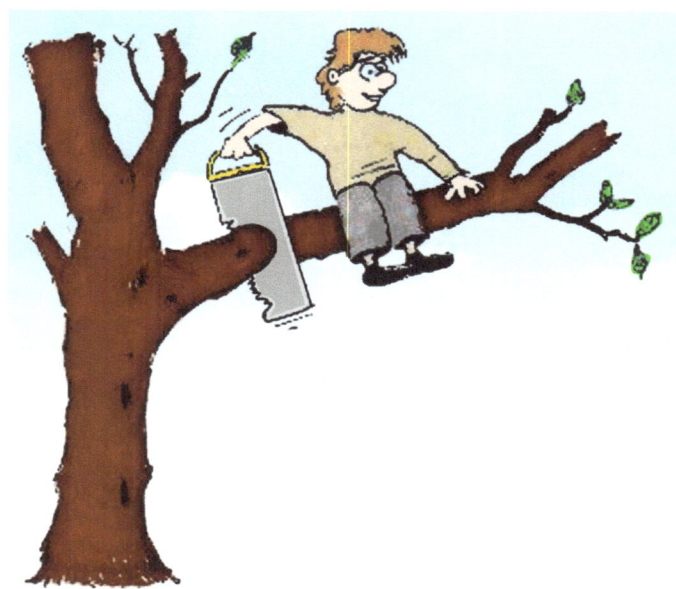

"You made me the loser I am today!"

Swallowing this one huge horse pill that the ONLY WAY OUT OF SUBSTANCE USE IS LEARNING TO SELF-CARE, and is the 'medicine' needed to prevent relapse.

Treatment providers must remain cognizant that substance users have a great difficulty learning this lesson even from their own experiences, and therefore have to become rather creative in helping teach this lesson. **As substance users seem not to learn well from the adverse results of their experiences, it is not then simply a matter of live and learn, but a drilling down more effectively to figure out what we need to learn in order to live, and then identifying and removing the obstacles that stand in the way of that learning.**

With proper training we can learn to use our prefrontal cortex like the steering wheel of a car to redirect our thoughts and feelings away from our anguish and turn us safely in the direction of our well being.

Our amygdala is our original built-in, 9-1-1 danger alarm detection system. Our prefrontal cortex functions as an override system: to detect prank calls and false alarms from the amygdala and to supervise and provide oversight to its responses.

While we need to keep our eyes open for the occasional lion, tiger, and bear, our survival these days may ultimately depend more on our ability to keep one eye on our own inner enemy—our amygdala—as well as on the amygdalas of others. One of the themes of this book is that we have yet to fully realize the threat and harm that comes from this relatively small area of our own brain.

As a result, we spend excessive amounts of our psychic energies in true Don Quixote-like fashion, jousting after windmills, effectively fighting the wrong and often imagined enemy. Mindfulness training teaches us that beyond staying away from brain and body toxins like cocaine, fentanyl, and alcohol, our worst enemy is not located outside ourselves in the drug, but in the inside part of our brain—the rather small, reckless part that impulsively and recklessly presses us to take these harmful substances into our bodies, all the while shouting from the rooftops:

"It's the only thing that works!"

Our amygdala too often functions like an improvised explosive device. We need to zoom in on this relatively small area of our brain's real estate to understand where our moodiness, irritability, boredom, distractibility, impulsivity, resentment, bitterness, rage, and self-hatred are sheltered. This is the area of our brain we need to learn about if we are to understand more fully why we are so often our own worst enemies.

Studies have shown that rage displays in a cat require no involvement of the cat's cortex

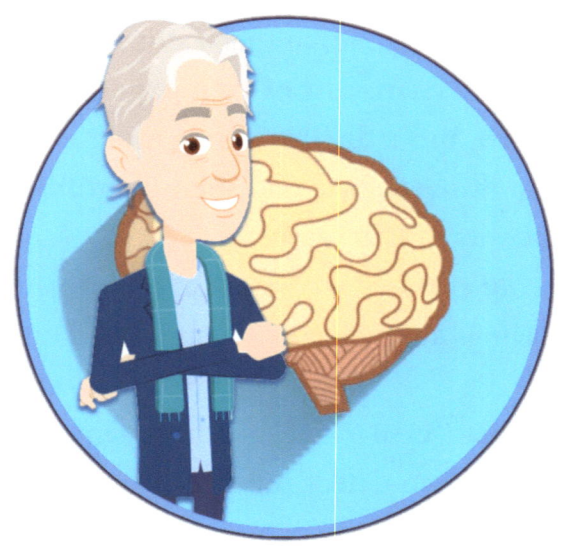

whatsoever. What if all of our negative human emotions, negative thinking and negative impulses involve little to none of our cortex? This would imply that we are truly dual-natured, and that our best and our higher nature sits right on top of our worst and lower nature. This would also imply that we do not have one mind, but two. It seems then that we unwisely turn to alcohol and substances to try to quiet the discomfort coming from our lower mind—our amygdala—not fully realizing that we are effectively pouring gasoline on a fire. When we use substances, the amygdala's flame might disappear for a moment, but by the next day the fire will be raging worse than ever.

With brain scans we can now 'see' what part of our brain is 'lighting up' when we are anxious, distressed, or angry, and what part of our brain lights up when we are peaceful and contented. Mindfulness teaches us not to leave the lights on in our mental basement—our amygdala—as it will just run up our mental utility bill and waste our psychic energy.

While most of our neuronal circuits function incredibly well on our behalf, some are really not that "smart"; they fire first and ask questions later, often generating decisions and behaviors that do not have our best interest at heart. We keep in mind the evolutionary perspective that our amygdala was designed to help us survive in the wilderness, where having a brain area devoted to keeping us hypervigilant may have meant the difference between life and death. This perspective is but small consolation, if today we remain so hypervigilant and so anxious that we can't get a good night's sleep and can't sit still.

We also can begin to appreciate how learning—even more so than instinct—and our capacity to learn, is now more directly linked to our survival. As we speak, thousands of human minds are focused and busy at work, stretching their collective learning,

The Evolutionary Perspective

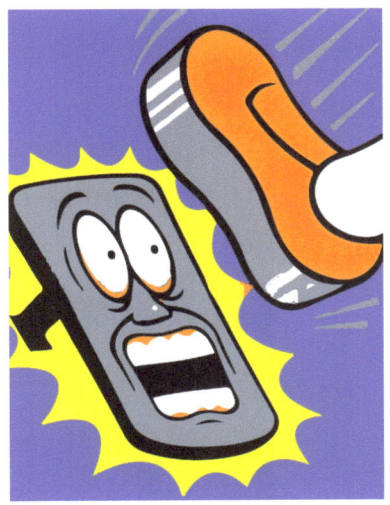 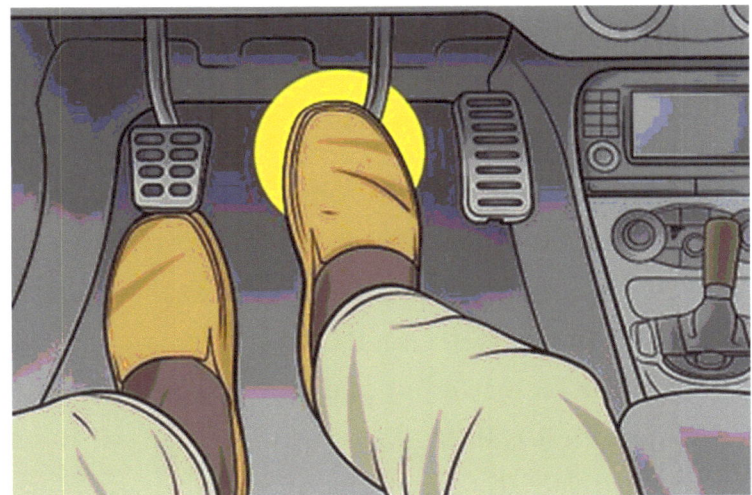

thinking and problem-solving circuits to design, develop, and implement a vaccine and treatments for the Corona Virus. The part of our brain that is capable of higher-level learning and higher-level thinking is what is especially unique about the human brain. Fortunately, we don't all have to become microbiologists in order to survive and thrive.

But it seems **we all do need to learn how to transcend the near-sighted automaticity of our lower psyche if we are to find our true measure of inner peace**, and steer a path away from self-harming thoughts, feelings and actions. Otherwise we will spend our psychic time and energy swatting at viruses with fly swatters, rather than gene-mapping and figuring out how to modify the viral genome in order to develop and produce an effective antidote.

Meanwhile, we must not lose sight of our equally pressing need to discover the **mental vaccine** and **mental antibodies** for our mental anguish, which if it leads us toward substance use, is also life-threatening and debilitating. Although neurons have been a part of existence for quite some time, they are unique cells, and they can do things that liver and heart cells can't do. The ability of neurons to make more and more connections with other neurons is at the heart of synaptic plasticity and learning and what makes the neuron unique.

New learning and new memories require new neurons with new connections. When we are haunted by horrible memories and faulty learnings, we can see that like an electrician having to replace, or at least circumvent, this older faulty tube wiring with new copper wiring.

Our brains are capable of doing this because we continue to make new neurons and can train these new neurons to make new connections to stop hanging out with the "old gang" and make some new neuron friends. It seems our neurons and neural circuits can function like the gas pedal or the brake of our cars, either activating our go circuits or our stop circuits, and it seems:

We come factory equipped as a very fast car with lousy brakes.

Mindfulness training helps us to change our mental brake lining so that we can more effectively stop any thought, feeling or action that might harm us. We learn to shift some of our attention to our speedometer to see how fast we are driving, and quickly slow down to avoid a ticket or worse. The braking mechanisms here are self-care and self-protection.

Each species has developed unique strategies to help ensure its survival. Our prefrontal cortex with its unique capacities for awareness, learning, problem-solving, and selectivity may as well be our most important survival tool. The prefrontal cortex is a tool that we can also strengthen and learn how to use more effectively. If we can learn to clean the lint screen off to help the dryer work more effectively, surely we can learn to identify and clear our minds of great quantities of mental lint that interfere with our brain's optimal functioning.

Mindfulness training teaches us to develop our prefrontal cortex's capacity to meta-think: to be aware of, reflect on, reappraise, and look at the price tag of every thought, feeling, impulse and behavior we have. When we do this, we become acutely aware of just how much mental stuff goes on between our ears that is simply not helpful, if not outright harmful.

When you are self-aware, it is you and your inner mental life that is the object of your attention. When you become aware of a higher and lower inner self, you realize you are watching an interesting mental tennis match, with the ball bouncing back and forth between two strong dueling opponents, each intensely focused on trying to exploit the other's weaknesses.

The Evolutionary Perspective

The amygdala is pushing to win the point quickly, while the prefrontal cortex is willing to rally for quite some time from the baseline, sensing that the amygdala's impatience will push it to hit the ball too hard to get the point over with. The amygdala's advantage is that is quicker, and quickness is a significant advantage in tennis.

However, the prefrontal cortex's advantage is that it is fully aware of its own strengths as well as its opponent's strengths and weaknesses. It pays careful attention to the amygdala's mounting frustration level. It knows that one or perhaps two carefully placed shots will likely press the amygdala to make a poor shot selection, sending the ball into the net out of bounds.

What is at stake for the tennis duel is winning a point or a game.

What is at stake for our mental duel is our well being, and even at times—our very lives.

Training our prefrontal cortex to take on and learn to dance differently with the amygdala is the essence of mindfulness training. Are you ready to put on your dancing shoes?

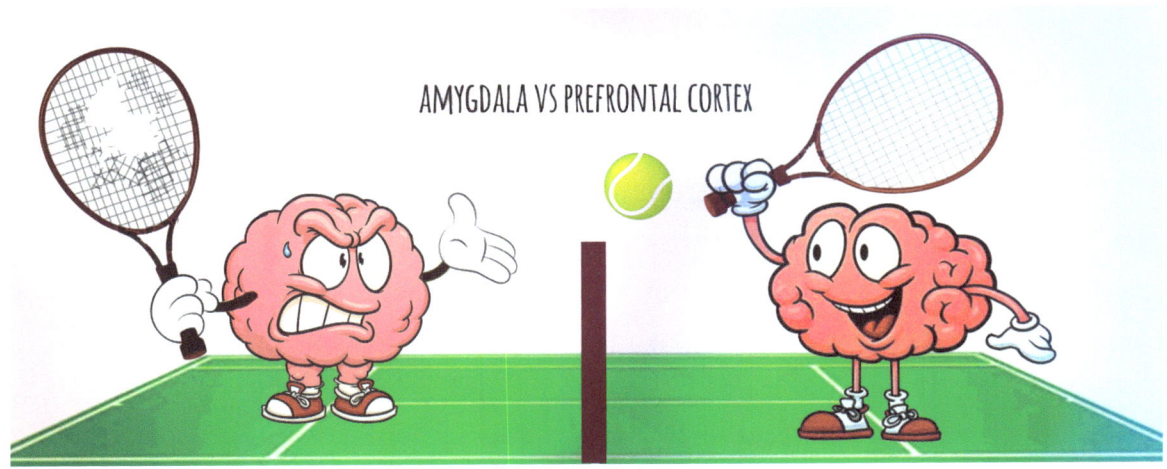

Mental Digestion

Now that we understand that our prefrontal cortex allows us to understand abstract concepts, we can drill down on some of the concepts that mindfulness introduces to us which help us understand ourselves better. For example, we understand from the study of human anatomy that our bodies have many organs providing different functions all working together at some level to help us survive and thrive. We readily understand that we have a gastrointestinal system that allows us to digest food, take in what we need, and also excrete that which is either toxic, a waste product, or simply not useful.

Mindfulness then, invites us to understand and utilize the concepts of mental digestion and mental indigestion. Mindfulness helps us to understand that **one of the essential mental functions of our brains is to help us digest our experiences**. The harsh reality however is that our brains do not digest upsetting experiences well. We all suffer with some degree of mental acid-reflux.

Because our brain comes factory-equipped with the human amygdala, we get irritated and excessively upset almost all the time, which only further adds to our mental and physical indigestion. When difficult-to-digest food lands in our stomachs, acid is released to help digest it. But we get ulcers when too much acid is released. When our mental brain attempts to digest toxic experiences, it immediately runs into many difficulties.

When we cannot seem to break the toxic experiences into smaller easier to digest pieces, our mind then repeatedly grinds and perseverates on what happened, and the mental glob of undigested muck has nowhere to go to be excreted, so it just sits there leaving us feeling crappy.

Our prefrontal cortex helps us to realize that unlike the physical body—which is indeed factory equipped to eliminate physical waste (urine, feces, sweat, exhale of CO_2), that there is no such factory-equipped mental waste excretion system. This is the kind of "yikes" realization that occurs when we more fully grasp the magnitude of the problem we are facing.

Mental Digestion

We can recall well when USA NASA astronauts discovered an explosion on their space shuttle and famously proclaimed to mission control: "Houston, we have a problem!" And, we also recall what we realized when the second plane crashed into the second World Trade Center tower on 9/11.

It is essential we realize that because we all possess an amygdala, we all have a ginormous human nature problem: **all human beings—all of us—are overloaded with mental waste** that oozes out of our amygdala, and we have **no built-in automatic excretion system to eliminate it**.

Our mission—should we choose to accept it— is to problem-solve and create ways to eliminate this mental waste. In the new pandemic lingo, learn to keep 6 feet of mental separation from it. If we can problem-solve how to get a man on the moon or how to remove physical waste from an astronaut suit, surely our problem-solving capabilities can come up with a solution for our mental waste.

Of course, it would have been much easier if our design included the automatic detection and removal of mental waste. But it seems that what evolution ingeniously designed for us is a brain area: our prefrontal cortex, that is equipped with the assessment and computational tools which enable us to find the solutions to the problems it did not fully anticipate.

The prefrontal cortex seems to possess all the tools we need to solve what has not been figured out in advance. When low oxygen levels in the water forced some aquatic life onto land to access the greater oxygen levels in the atmosphere, it took millions of years of rather remarkable evolutionary engineering to roll out the first lung prototypes.

The first reptiles stepping onto land realized they too had a ginormous problem. The genetic mutations that created lungs allowed those species of new land dwellers to survive, while the others needed to either return to the water or perish. One stroke of evolutionary engineering genius was to equip our species with the capacity to realize exactly what it needed to develop to survive in a new, life-threatening circumstance and to give it the wherewithal to make those adaptations without having to wait for a genetic modification bailout.

Our prefrontal cortex is that feature built-in to our brain that allows us to adapt and not end up on the perish heap. Our mission is to get this part of our brain cranking! Keep in mind, no other living species that exists now, or that has ever existed, has been aware that it possesses a brain, never mind been aware of the tools within the brain's toolbox. Mindfulness training teaches where to find and select the right mental screwdriver, as well as where to find the one or two screws that run around loose in all of us.

The irony is that we all have troubling thoughts and feelings. At times, we feel we don't belong, we think we are defective, and we consider ourselves to be misfits. None of these thoughts or feelings are true or accurate. What is true is that we all have a built-in negativity generator spewing these negative thoughts and feelings out in mass quantities. All human beings have this built-in negativity generator. Since we all have an amygdala, and since the amygdala spews negativity, we now better understand the mindfulness dictum: "**I have an amygdala, therefore I suffer!**"

On the flip side of the coin, it is also true that all people, by possession of our human brain, are also in possession of a remarkable prefrontal cortex, and therefore also have wonderful thoughts, inspired ideas, feelings and impulses.

Most human beings discover that they have an **overactive amygdala, juxtaposed to an underdeveloped prefrontal cortex**. But this realization can be very helpful to us, as it urges us to be less preoccupied with other people's imbalances and focus instead on assessing and rectifying our own.

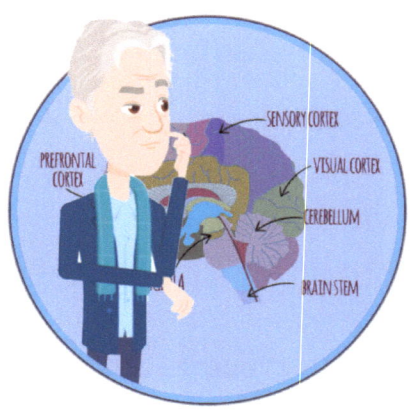

Learning to be aware of one's amygdala, while not being hijacked by it, as well as learning how to more fully access the tools and fruits of our prefrontal cortex becomes our focus.

We also have to learn to recognize those who are clueless regarding how to manage and regulate their amygdala, and more wisely choose to not make these people our life partners. We should also keep a safe distance from them in other settings,

Mental Digestion

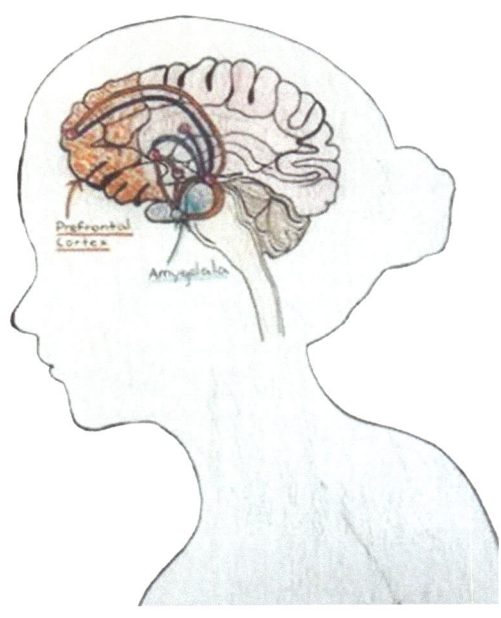

even if they include family members. Learning about our brain helps us to realize that we, our abusers, our parents, kids, siblings, friends, neighbors, and every human being is in the same boat by having an amygdala..

The amygdala is a relatively tiny brain module that is our weakest and most challenging brain link—a leaking hole in our otherwise fabulous boat. The best of our humanity will drain out of the hole, unless and until we lean to plug the hole and learn to navigate keeping one eye on our destination, and the other on the status of the leak.

Fortunately, our amygdala is surrounded by other rather fabulous brain modules which can function as a team to limit the amount of havoc the amygdala can create.

One of these brain modules, the prefrontal cortex, is quite large and is quite capable (especially with training) of effectively arm-wrestling the amygdala, and providing effective leadership and amygdala oversight.

The next major problem we must realize is that the human amygdala is actually a mental waste maker. It not only doesn't contribute to the elimination of mental waste, but also actually produces the bulk of it. Our amygdala soils its own nest, so to speak. Our amygdala is our mental polluter. The amygdala is the seat of fight or flight responses and therefore is the seat of our aggression and fear. When a primate's amygdala is activated, it directs its aggression outwardly toward scoring a potential meal, or defending and protecting itself and its babies. When humans get aggressive, we alternate between directing aggression outwardly and inwardly.

It is this inward directed aggression that is at the center of our negative self-thinking and impulses to self-injure. The human brain is a remarkable success story. However, the amygdala section of the human brain is not particularly remarkable, and does not, in my view, compare favorably to the amygdala of other species.

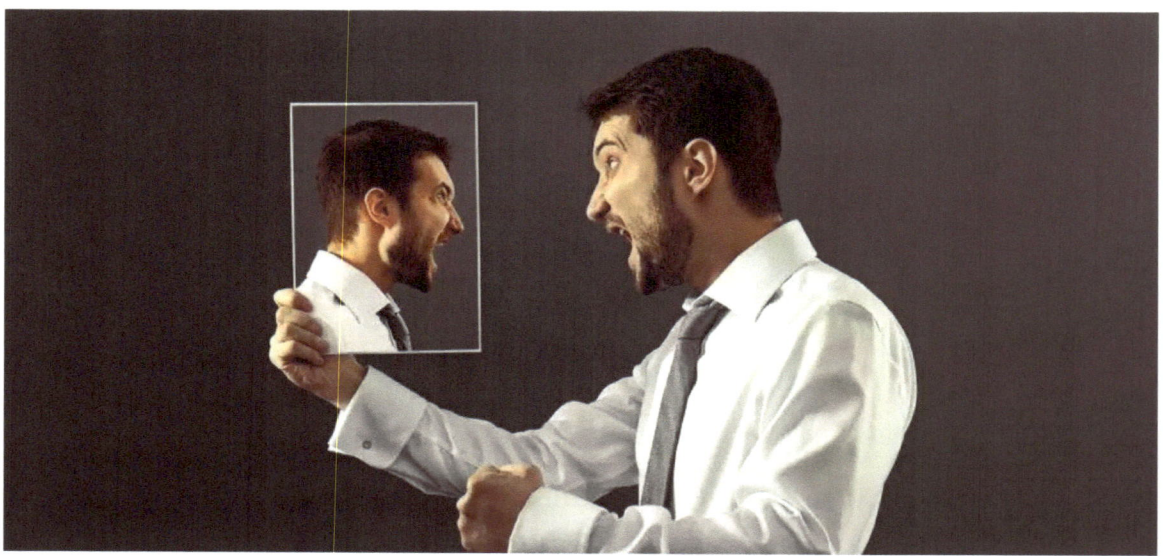

If we did not have a prefrontal cortex to help override our amygdala, we would be in even worse shape. With mindfulness training we learn to become more and more aware of our self-directed negativity and the various guises it comes in. It is especially evident in our negative self-thinking. Let's face it: If you have said to yourself once: "How could I be so stupid?"—you have said it a thousand times!

Humans are the only living entity that is in the self-directed negativity business, and there can be no doubt: we all excel at it. Mindfulness teaches us that almost all of our self-directed negativity is wasteful.

The oracle of Delphi directed us to 'Know yourself", while the oracle of mindfulness helps us become aware of just how often we actually say 'no' to, ourselves and just how counter-productive that is to do.

If you throw a dog a Frisbee and it misses, it doesn't waste a moment thinking negatively about itself, but simply wags its tail and readies itself, playfully and expectantly for the next throw. But if a human being drops the Frisbee they will become mortified and will immediately think: "I'm such a spaz!" and presume that anyone watching will be thinking the same! It seems this self-directed negativity is the price we pay for having the most advanced brain on the evolutionary market. Mindfulness training teaches us how to lower the cost of this mental utility bill, just as an Amazon

Firestick can help us lower our cable bill. The human brain is unique in allowing us a significant amount of hardware and software updates.

We need to use the tools of our prefrontal cortex to remedy this negativity problem. The mental blades of awareness, realization, selectivity, and conscious purposeful attention shift to redress this problem, enabling us to get to the part of our brain that houses our higher mind which is free of amygdala pollution.

We learn that we need to climb out of the amygdala basement and go by any means possible to the higher level of the prefrontal cortex. How do we maneuver from one part of our brain to another? Whatever way your creative, higher mind can devise! Call an Uber, climb the staircase, use the escalator or elevator, scale the wall, jump up, use a rope, call a friend, or hitchhike!

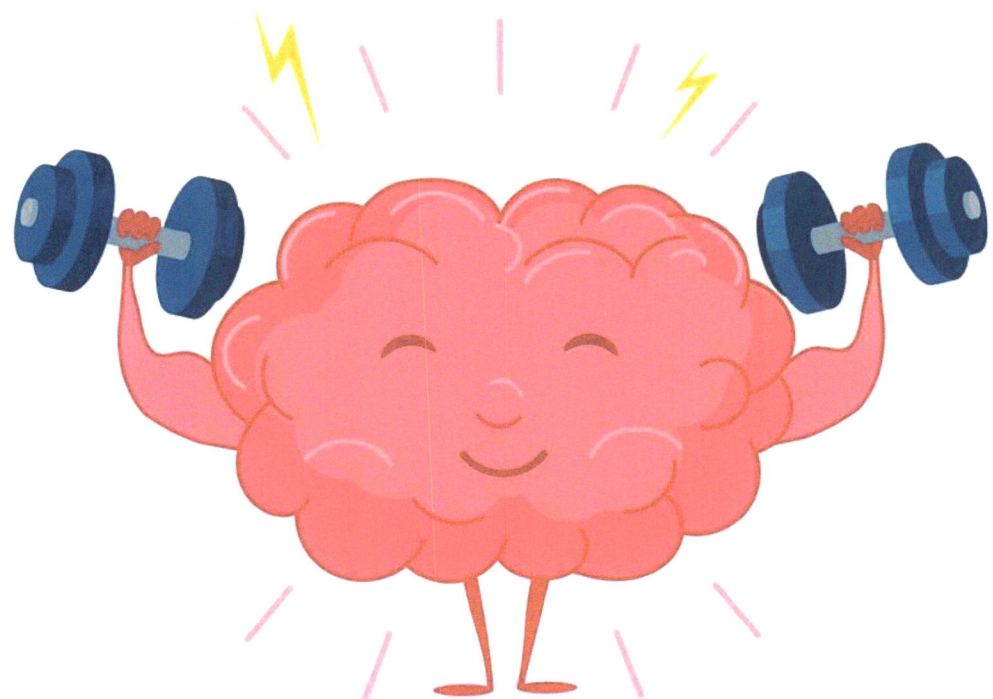

Do whatever you need to do to get out of your mental basement with the proviso that what you do does not in the end, make your basement any bigger or stronger. While alcohol and substances may give a few moments of reprieve from your flooded basement, by the time you wake up the next morning, your basement is flooded at least six inches deeper (that is, if you are still alive).

Our prefrontal cortex can function like a sump pump to pump the unwanted water out of our flooded basement. However, it functions at its best when it is meta-thinking. From a creative, landscaping perspective, this means it is devising ways to divert the water from the outside so that it doesn't flood the basement in the first place!

The key approach that mindfulness training teaches us for getting out of our basement is the **conscious shifting of our attention**. This is analogous to learning to use a stick shift. You learned to listen closely to the sound of the engine, which would indicate by its loud sound when it was time to shift to another gear. Mindfulness training teaches us that we are almost always in the wrong gear, and that the mental noise we need to listen to is the noise of our own discomfort.

Most of our physical waste products have a smell that accompanies them which helps us to remember they are indeed meant to be eliminated. Moreover, we never identify ourselves with these products we flush down the toilets.

Mindfulness training is required, in large part, because we have to train ourselves to be aware of the smell of what AA refers to as our stinking thinking. It seems we also have to devise mental toilets to help flush the negative thoughts, feelings, memories and impulses that form such a yucky, dirty, cloudy, film on our mental windshields. This film is typically most noticeable when we wake up and when we try to fall asleep.

Mindfulness training is required to help separate a sense of ourselves from these stinking thoughts, otherwise we don't realize that we are simply having these stinking thoughts about ourselves such as: I am a failure, defective, a misfit—and having these thoughts does not make them true. Moreover, the awareness of having these kinds of thoughts, which itself is a higher level of thinking, is actually quite helpful and has a wonderful aroma to it; while the baseline thoughts themselves do indeed stink.

MENTAL DIGESTION

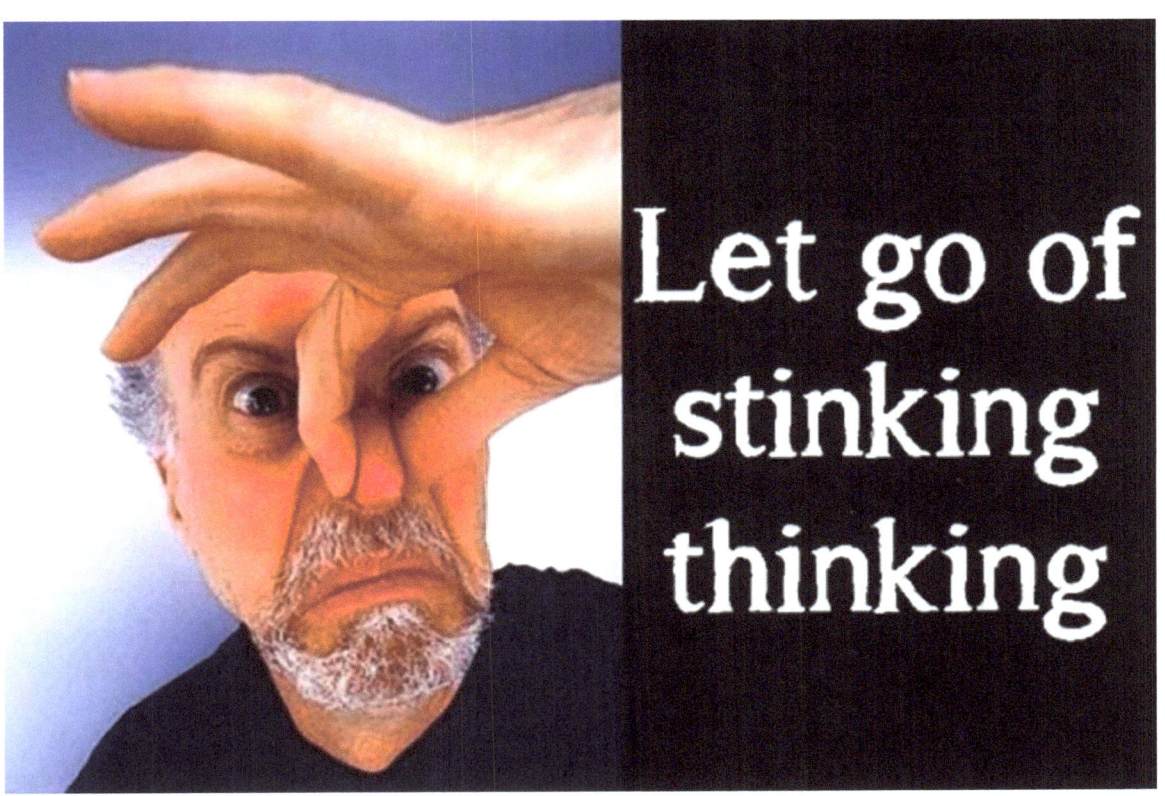

This awareness operates at a higher level of our mental capacities, is sweet-smelling, and from the higher perch of our meta-thinking, we can look down on, oversee, and eventually learn to be amused by, our lower-level stinking thinking.

We become empowered and liberated when we combine this oversight with the compassionate awareness that all human beings spend way too much time unnecessarily drinking from, and bathing in, this polluted stream. We can imagine that our higher cognition emerged from the building blocks of lower cognition, and perhaps like fishermen, we have to throw a lot of thoughts, feelings and impulses back before we find the ones that we want to reel in.

Or we can imagine that some of our thoughts and feelings have no nutritional value whatsoever, and are but a mere waste product of the thinking-feeling production system itself. Whether what is on the line is too small, or actually toxic, we are called upon to **pay careful attention to what we have hooked, and always remember that we are the catcher and not what we catch**.

This awareness of and our separation from our thoughts and feelings and our identification with them, is the essence of a new enlightened understanding we can develop about ourselves and is captured in this book's title: *Me, Myself, and My Amygdala*.

Our meta-thoughts help us to become more aware of these lower-level thoughts; that while we have these thoughts, we are not these thoughts. Our meta-thinking is our positive, useful, beneficial thoughts.

It is the part of our thinking that allows us to think about ourselves with compassionate reflection, and to become aware of and free ourselves from our rampant negative subjectivity.

Human beings are judgmental about themselves and others, more so than any other living entity. Being judgmental is vintage lower-level thinking.

Being judgmental is about as useful to us as having an appendix. It seems like the only function the appendix serves is to become inflamed and have to be surgically removed.

But the level of our mental faculty that is meta (above, higher) to being judgmental is our ability to make distinctions. We make distinctions by becoming more discerning, which allows us to pay closer attention to the difference between one thing and another.

A mother and her baby must be able to recognize one another amongst the noisy and distracting herd or flock and be able to make subtle distinctions in sound, appearance, or smell to do so.

The survival value of making distinctions is evident. We can really benefit by making distinctions. Our ability to discern—to make meaningful distinctions between one thing and another—is a beneficial higher cognitive function which we need more of.

This higher ability allows us to discern when we are being judgmental, as discernment is a kind of awareness that can become quite focused—like zooming in with a camera lens. We can learn to cut off our judgmentalism—like cutting the gristle off a piece of steak.

If we don't train ourselves to make the important distinctions between our normative stinking thinking and our meta-thinking, we conclude that these normative thoughts are facts:

"I am a failure!"

"I screw everything up!"

"I'm a huge disappointment!"

We become hijacked by and identify with our stinking thinking. If these thoughts were physical in nature and were accompanied by a nasty smell, we would not hesitate to flush them. But because they are mental in nature, we have to train ourselves to separate ourselves from them.

Although, we do not have the developed sense of smell that dogs have, we do have the capacity to learn to sniff things out. With training and practice, we soon can be sniffing out and confiscating the suitcase-filled loads of stinking thoughts that fill our minds daily.

We can begin to imagine that we can install a kind of **mental Homeland Security Detector**, and place all our thoughts, feelings and impulses on our newly devised **mental metal detector**. All that doesn't pass metal is confiscated and thrown away.

Brian L. Ackerman, M.D.

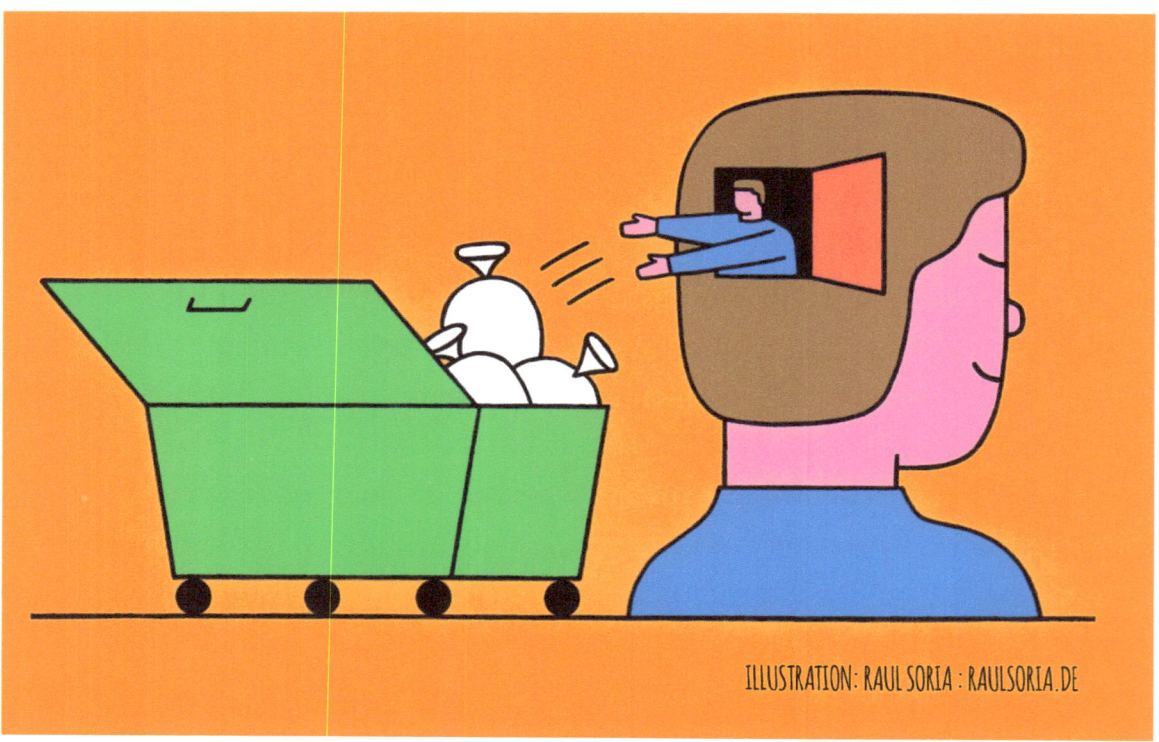

ILLUSTRATION: RAUL SORIA : RAULSORIA.DE

Mindfulness introduces the concept of **mental toxicity** and helps us to see our negative thoughts and feelings, impulsivity, and harmful and counter-productive behavior as manifestations of this toxicity. It also teaches us how to utilize the pre-frontal cortex to problem solve what we must learn to do about this **toxic mental waste.**

Given that there is no built-in elimination mechanism—no excretion system for mental waste, no lungs for the mind, so to speak—we must find a way to both identify the waste, and deliberately and intentionally develop the means to cart it away and free ourselves from its accumulation and toxic effects.

The Purpose-Driven Mindfulness

There are a number of different approaches to mindfulness that are available. The method that I have developed, I call the purpose-driven mindfulness. Many meditation and mindfulness programs can come across as somewhat vague about their purpose. In general, they invite us to take time to pause, quiet the mental noise, and to relax. Indeed, these are wonderful and useful things to do. Most of our lives, we run around like chickens with our heads cut off, so we can intuitively understand the benefit of the "Don't just do something, sit there!" approach. However, I see the purpose of mindfulness as going much further than sitting there and relaxing. In the purpose-driven mindfulness, the focal point is less to relax, but to learn—especially about our human brain.

Learning about our brain is one of the most direct routes to learning about oneself and others. When we learn about the brain, we learn that when we are anxious and stressed, **only a very small portion of our brain is in that 'stressed' state, while the rest of the brain is cool as a cucumber**. When we learn about the brain, we learn we can relax not by trying to get the tiny stressed part of our brain to calm down, but by actively and intentionally stepping into the larger regions of our brain that are already quite peaceful. When it's raining out, it's much easier and effective to step into a building that is already protected, then to start a rain dance to get the rain to stop falling.

Or if you find yourself in a room where the AC has been off, why not go to the next room where the AC is on and working rather than turning on the AC and staying in the uncomfortable room until it cools down? We can think of the various brain modules like rooms in our homes.

The prefrontal cortex is always air-conditioned and comfortable, but we know we have stepped into the amygdala room the moment we become uncomfortable. It almost always raining in our amygdala and in Seattle, and almost never rains in our prefrontal cortex or Aruba.

While I have met many people who, oddly enough, don't seem that interested in understanding themselves, I have never met anyone who is not really curious about their brain. This curiosity about our brain then becomes the starting point to self-understanding.

The purpose of mindfulness training is to help us learn enough about our brains so that we can **redirect the greater part of our psychic energies toward the intelligent pursuit of our well-being**. Like meditation and yoga, meditation training teaches us the importance of getting out of our noisy minds.

But once out, mindfulness teaches us to actually go back into our brain so we can access and utilize the best part of our brain: our upper mind where our intelligence, creativity, capacity for redirection, and best selves await us and are calling out for our return.

We learn about our brain's purpose: an organ devoted to helping us survive as well as thrive. And we learn that most of our brain, while serving many essential functions, contributes very little to our psychological sense of ourselves. We learn that although we have many brain modules, that there are only two brain areas which drive our psychological sense of ourselves, and these two areas are almost always diametrically opposed in their agendas.

It is of no wonder that **we are of two minds about everything!**

We are not a singular self, but rather we have dueling, conflicting selves, derived from very different locations in our brain. We learn about the characteristics of these two conflicting mental modules.

Our lower module is quick, impulsive, self-injurious, negative, and remarkably short-sighted. It was designed to be on high-alert for survival in the wild; while our higher module is a bit slower, more thoughtful and reflective, and delights in many higher-level distinctions, that allow us to patiently but deliberately problem-solve. It also helps us to make wiser self and other-caring choices and decisions, and to look beyond imagined immediate rewards to our future safety and to the well-being of us and others. Our lower module was designed to keep us on high alert, with sensors on high gain to pick up even a whiff of danger.

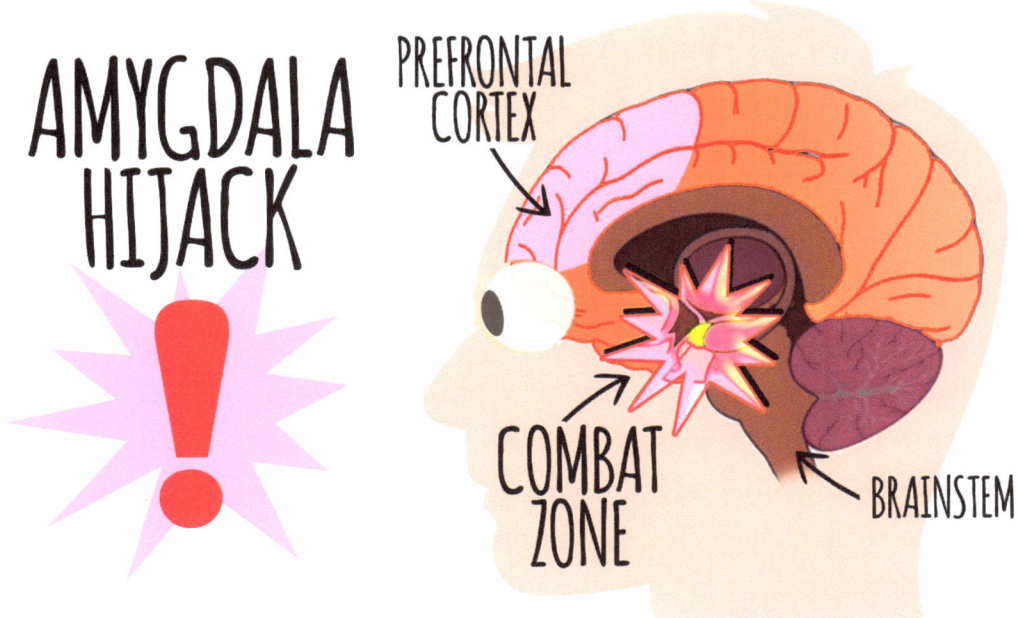

Our higher module guides us to our well-being, our joy, our gladness, and our delight to be alive. Our higher module, unique to our human brain, allows us to be aware of the lower module. The higher module is educable and be can be trained to take all that emanates from the lower module with a grain of salt and restrain, and if need be, override the lower module's impulses and preoccupations.

We learn that even when we are feeling overwhelmed by anxiety, only our amygdala and its immediate connections are 'anxious', while all the other brain modules actually remain quite peaceful.

Our higher module allows us to be aware of having a brain, and even more specifically, allows us to be aware of where in the brain the **module of awareness** is located. This same higher module allows us to make distinctions between our higher, true purposes, and our lower purposes. The lower purpose of eating, for example, is to make the discomfort of our hunger pains go away; the higher purpose of eating is to select wisely the food we ingest which will be most beneficial and least harmful. If we attend exclusively to our lower purpose, fries and ice cream may be chosen as we rush to put any quality of gas in the tank—and sugary, tasty, food suffices.

But if we attend to our higher purpose, and we pause to consider just how much we want and need our engine to last, fruit and spring water might be the more self-caring and satisfying choices.

Mindfulness training reminds us to be aware of, and stay connected to, our higher purposes as often as we can. We select healthy foods to stay alive and thrive in order that we can lead a meaningful and fulfilling life, care for others, carry out our life's mission, spare ourselves and others avoidable pain and injury, and extract the most we can out of our limited lifetime. Our higher module, the prefrontal cortex, is the only part of the brain capable of tuning in to these higher purposes.

When we study the brain, we can see how purpose-driven it is as a whole, and how purpose-driven the individual modules within the brain are. The brain stem's purpose is to regulate oxygen, glucose, and body temperature etcetera. The purpose of the vision model is so we can see, the auditory module so we can hear, the language module so we can speak, understand, and be understood, the cerebellum module so we can maintain physical balance, the motor cortex, so we can move our arms and legs and the sensory cortex so we can touch, taste, and feel.

The purpose of the prefrontal cortex is so that we can see the big picture, see the potential benefit or adverse impact down the road of something we are considering, stay above the fray, plan and choose a course of action wisely and intelligently, make executive decisions, grasp more abstract concepts like love and higher purpose, remain aware of and cultivate the growing and aspiring spirit inside us, and purposely and actively shift our attention, away from our many distractions and preoccupations. This allows us to become more laser-focused on that which truly matters, and to strategize and plan how to bring us closer to what matters most.

A tenet of mindfulness is that **our well-being is tied to the degree to which we are aligned with our higher purpose**. But what is our higher purpose? We can become clearer about what our higher purpose is, by first becoming clearer about what it is not!

Clearly the purpose of having the best brain on the evolutionary market is not to have us consumed by negative thoughts and feelings about ourselves. And without a brain, we would have none of these.

The Purpose-Driven Mindfulness

With mindfulness training, we learn to compassionately witness our thoughts and feelings. We humbly discover just how many of them are negative, and how effortlessly a part of our brain produces this negativity. We literally can do this with our eyes closed!

We can understand that one purpose of our brain is survival, while another purpose is the intelligent pursuit of our well-being. We can also understand that areas of our brain devoted to these somewhat different purposes may often be out of alignment, if not in outright conflict. Mindfulness training can help us be more aware of this misalignment, and not to get so frustrated with ourselves because of it, but instead to make more purposeful adjustments accordingly.

Mindfulness calls upon us to wrap our mental arms around this negative productivity, to begin to make sense of it, and to learn how to best relate to and dispose of its productions. We might say about an orange tree that its purpose is to grow, produce leaves, blossoms, oranges, fragrance, and seed for the next generation. When an orange tree is achieving its purpose, we say it is thriving. But for us humans, what is our comparable higher purpose?

What do humans look like, and what are they feeling when they are thriving?

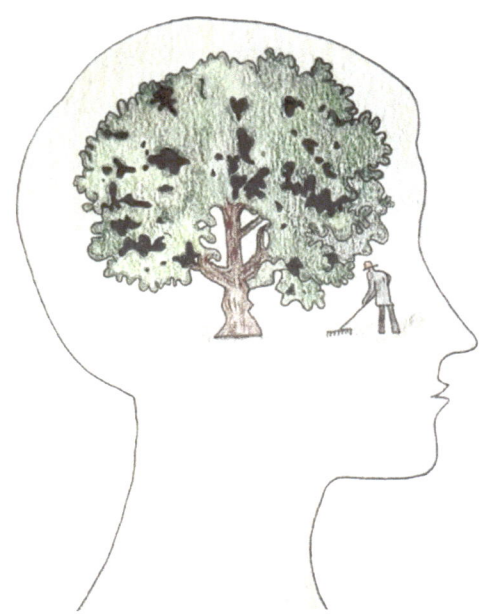

We can understand these two truths: that the purpose of the human brain is not to produce negative thoughts, feelings and impulses, while recognizing that, nonetheless, it, in fact, produces a lot of them. We can consider the model of dual productions of an automobile factory—producing both cars that are quite useful, as well as producing smoke that is quite toxic—to help us understand the difference between positive purposeful production, and adverse undesired, unintended co-production. Or, we can return to the model of physical digestion that both produces the energy we need to live, as well the waste that needs to be eliminated. We can also begin to appreciate the irony that without our advanced brain, we would have none of these mentally toxic thoughts, feelings, or impulses.

Much of what we remember troubles us. We often see ourselves in a negative light. These mental functions: remembering, and the many ways we imagine ourselves, can cut both in positive, beneficial ways—or negative and harmful ways.

Much of life exists with no brain. Amongst brains of many living species, past and present, the human brain is rather unique. We can ask how does having a mental life that we are aware of aid our survival? The following vignette will help us to understand the survival advantage of having a mental life that we are aware of:

A human walking in the woods comes across a rattlesnake. The human amygdala 'thinks" fight or flight. Either fight: pick up a stick and kill the snake, or flight: run like Hell. The snake, however, is factory-equipped with motion detectors so either of these movements—picking up the stick or running would activate the snake to bite. However, with an internal mental life, we could pause to consider what the intentions of the snake are and where it might go if we just became silent. Perhaps it will just mosey on?

One clear survival advantage of our inner mental life is to give us more choices and see beyond the limited choices the amygdala offers. Perhaps then the iconic image of a meditator sitting in a yoga position, pausing, quietly breathing, can be enhanced by an image of being in a self-huddle where the pause and the quiet is for the purpose of thinking with greater clarity of the next intelligent move—which at times, is not to move at all!

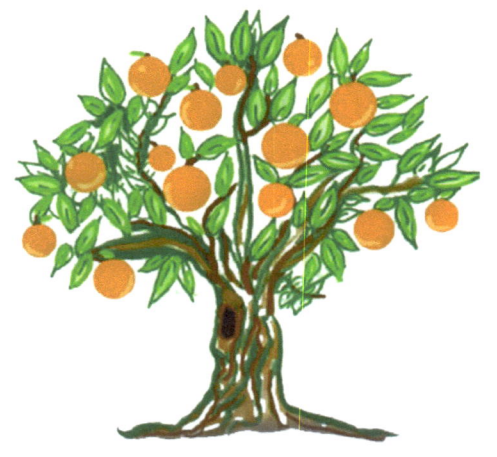

One of the insights of meditation-based practices is to help us realize that our constant doing often becomes so compulsive that we become lost when we have nothing to do.

Learning to just be in the moment, peacefully enjoying being aware of our breathing

The Purpose-Driven Mindfulness

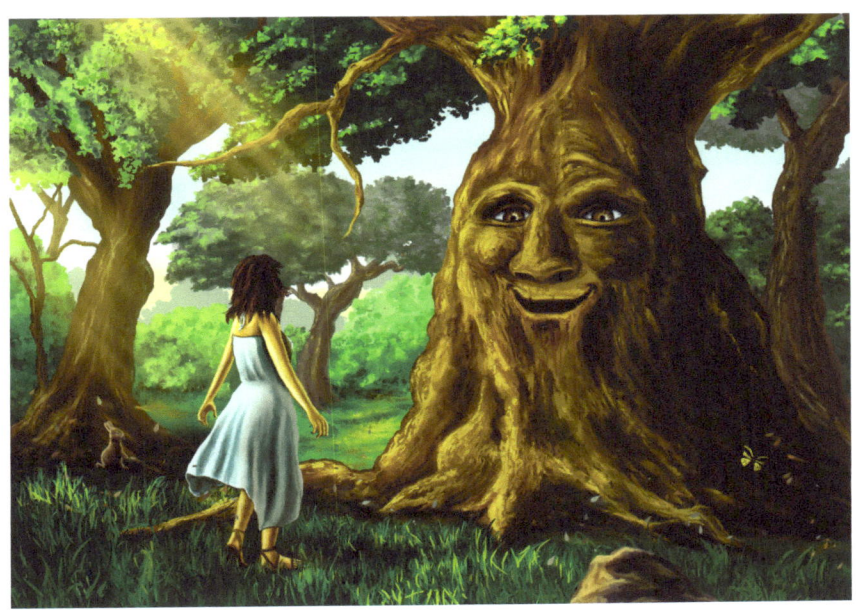

and being alive is central to this approach. Mindfulness training then invites us to learn to be able to return to our doing so that whatever we are doing or not doing, we learn how to do it in a more enlightened way—whether that be eating, showering, or paying attention to the effect of what we say and do on others. We also pay particular attention to the effect on ourselves of what is whirling around in our mind.

Perhaps another advantage is to help us become aware of and learn how to constrain the many ways in which our inner mental life is actually disadvantageous. Most of life exists without a brain. A lot of life exists with a rather rudimentary one.

To help us better understand and appreciate how we benefit from having these added features, I offer the following dialog between a human and a tree.

Human to Tree:

"I must confess; I have **tree envy.** I look at you and you seem so peaceful and contented. You seem rooted and down to earth. You don't seem the least bit distracted and you are in no hurry. You seem to know your purpose and remain focused on achieving it. You seem focused on growing taller, growing leaves, blooming buds, producing fruit, fragrance and seed, and you don't seem to waste a moment comparing yourself to any other tree. You seem blessed to be unaware that you are a tree, or that you are vulnerable to death, or that dogs use you for target practice, or that humans use you for firewood and timber. I envy the way you are living; simply content to be alive, taking adversity in stride, not aspiring to be anything more than being and becoming the healthiest and best tree you can be. Your way of life I can only dream about."

Tree to Human:

"I really do understand your perspective, and, yes, being a tree without being plagued by a single negative thought or feeling, and just thoroughly enjoying being alive, celebrating life, and celebrating being alive is without a doubt the best experience ever! It is at the heart of what I believe the East calls **Nirvana!** However, I must confess: I have **human envy**, as I would give my right limb to truly know what it means to be alive, to truly know that I am a tree, to be curious what kind of tree, and even to know that I will not live forever. I would give my left limb to communicate verbally, to love, to move, to dance, to sing and to comprehend even a thimbleful of what you can comprehend about yourselves and about the universe.

So, here is my challenge question to you: Given that you have this rather amazing human brain that I don't, can't you learn how to utilize more effectively its rather remarkable features and use your capacity to learn, to devise some way to take your negative thoughts and feelings with a grain of salt? Even though I'm a tree, I never think of myself as a sap! It seems that if you were able to learn to do this, you could come really come close to realizing the incredibly peaceful, contented, and focused way of living that you imagine that I enjoy, as well as realize all the additional amazing experiences that are made possible, exclusively to you, and optimize the best of both your world and mine?"

With mindfulness, we can learn to be more aware of, and ultimately amused by, the part of our brain that interferes with our higher purpose.

We cannot teach the lower brain how to be peaceful; it is just not built that

way—but we can learn, to not allow it to define us, govern us, or keep us from recognizing our loving, kind-hearted, funny and fun-loving, joyous and peaceful higher nature, or keep us from bringing forth our unique contributions to the world.

Humans are noted for their rather wide range of thoughts and feelings. However, what truly makes humans unique is our capacity to be aware of this entire mental thought and feeling panorama, and then learn to be more selective from its wide-ranging contents—like what to pay attention to. We make similar kinds of selections daily when we change the channels of our televisions and radios.

Mindfulness training helps us to be more aware of and choose the better of our mental channels. To have inner peace, we must learn to stop watching and listening to the anxiety channel and the depression network!

Darwin wrote about the survival of the fittest, which largely had to do with physical attributes and physical abilities. Mindfulness opens the door to be developing our mental fitness. Our survival may depend much more on our mental abilities—which are open for development.

Our very survival may depend on our mental ability to become aware of and quarantine ourselves from our destructive impulses, our ability to understand problems and solve them, and our mental ability to become mentally fit and **learn to shift our time, energy and attention away from counter-productive pre-occupations, to more fruitful endeavors.**

Perhaps we are moving in the direction of the **Survival of the Aware-est**. Mindfulness can be seen as a tool we can learn to utilize to help us not only survive but thrive. Our prefrontal cortex evolved to help us pay attention to that which is most important, and to help us extract from our experience that which is most relevant and useful toward helping us achieve our higher purpose. Humans don't produce oranges, but the fruit of our humanity is our capacity for love, kindness, compassion, as well as creative and constructive problem-solving.

We can use mindfulness to be more aware of what is ripening inside us and to help us create the internal mental climate to facilitate this ripening.

We can also **learn just how much of our discomfort is created from within**, and

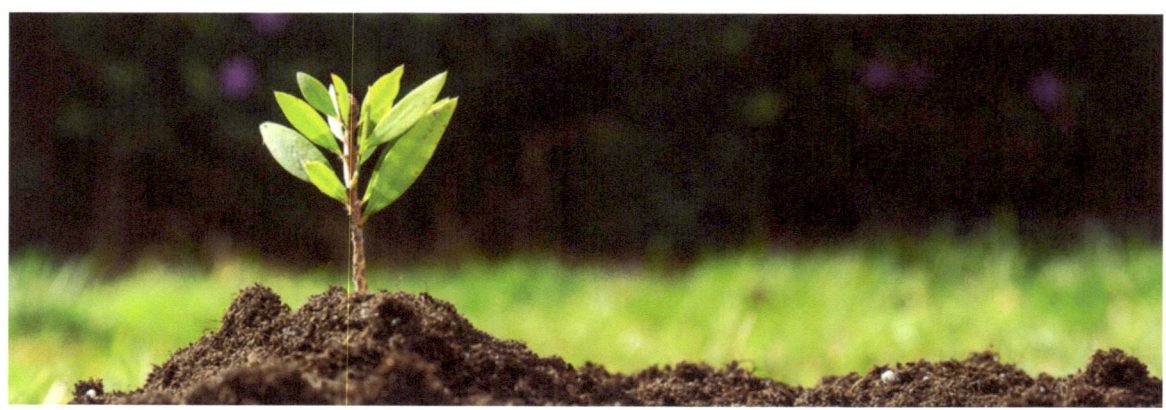

to insert higher level associations in the crucial milliseconds between our triggers and our responses, allowing us to access and sustain more positive mental states of inner peace and serenity, while learning to avoid the built-in pot holes of our negativity and lower-self preoccupations.

As a result, anger, negative thoughts and feelings, and other harmful impulses flash like mental fireflies for moments—not hours or days.

Moreover, we strengthen our capacity to shift gears out of the swampy mosquito-ridden states, to our upper screened-in porches where we can **realign with our higher purpose**, feel more alive—more illuminated, open-minded, wise, and joyful—and free ourselves from the parts of our nervous system that would otherwise hijack us.

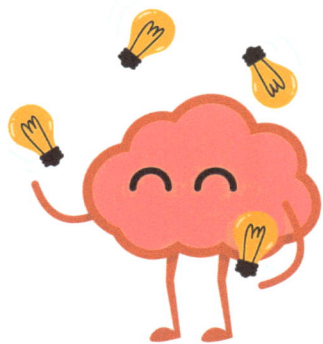

Excremation Points

If we step back to see how things that are alive keep themselves alive, we will notice that even for a tiny single-celled organism, there is a membrane that functions as a filter, allowing into the interior of the cell that which is needed, while at the same time exporting out of the interior of the cell all that has not become toxic waste material. This filtration mechanism is essential for survival. In humans, urea is made in the liver when protein is broken down and passed out of the body in the urine. If the kidney's filtration is not working properly, nitrogen builds up in our blood stream and can makes us quite sick. If not removed, we can die.

A BUN blood test measures the level of blood urea nitrogen in the body, and is an indicator of how well our kidneys are functioning. Our kidneys are essential filters, retaining water and minerals, while excreting urea. If our kidneys fail, we need to go on kidney (renal) dialysis, so that a machine can mechanically filter out the urea for us.

If we look at how the human body is organized, **our organs are functioning as overlapping filters.** Like the membrane of a single cell, our organs filter and help bring inside us what is needed; proteins, nutrients and oxygen inside every cell, all while excreting outside of us that which has become toxic.

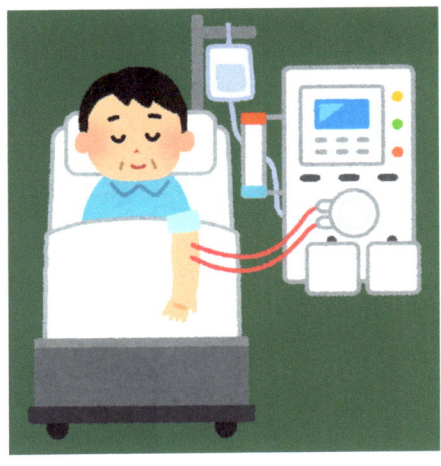
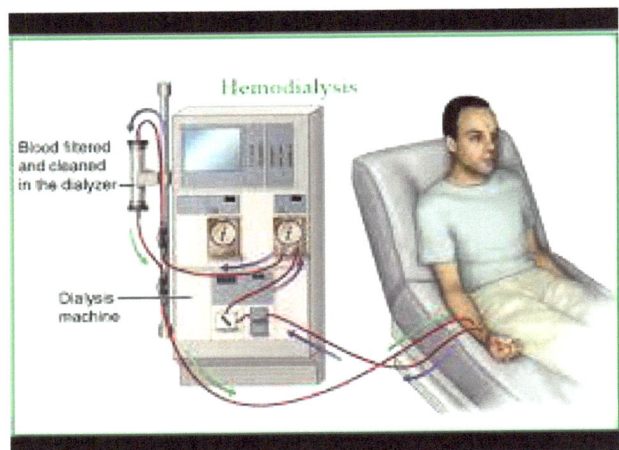

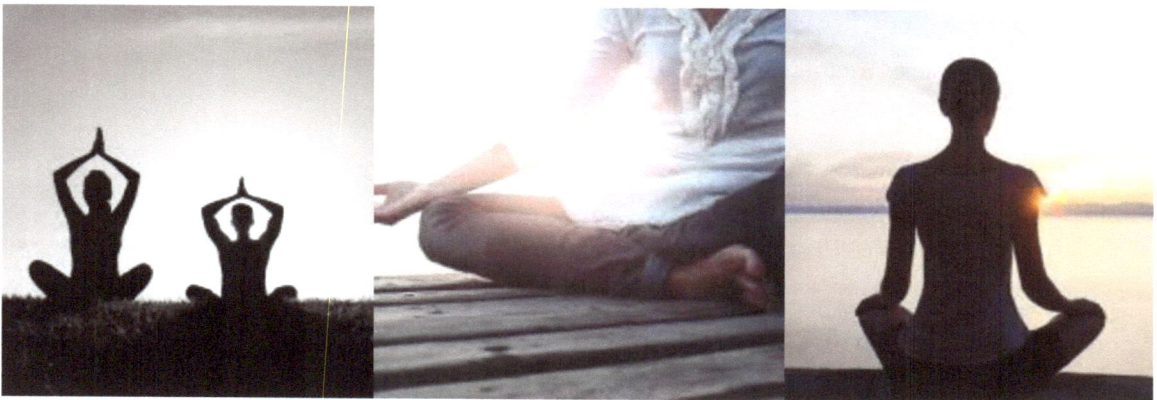

Our gastrointestinal system is filtering the food we need, and that which is not beneficial or which has been used and is now toxic, is excreted.

The most graceful filtration system we have in our body and the iconic image of meditation and mindfulness is breathing. Twelve times a minute, silently, the lining of our lungs extracts oxygen from the universe while excreting back into the universe carbon dioxide—which makes the trees happy but will make us sick and die if we cannot get rid of it. During your meditation practice when you are paying attention to your breath, I encourage you to be thinking about this **fundamental exchange and filtration that is going on between you and the universe,** as well as how good it feels to breathe. This is especially helpful when you are feeling like a misfit or that you don't belong. Your breathing and moment-by-moment exchange with the universe is **proof positive that you absolutely do fit and do belong**.

The meditation adage is that when you become frenzied, return to your breath and begin again.

Another important concept I introduce in mindfulness training is **mental waste**.

Our brains produce many incredible capabilities such as our capacity for love, joy, caring, thoughtfulness, creativity, problem solving etcetera, but it seems **our brains also produce mental waste products by the boat load**—chock full of negative thoughts, negative feelings, negative impulses, negative attitudes and negative memories.

Let's take a moment now to understand the different between the purpose of a product and the production of a by-product.

Excremation Points

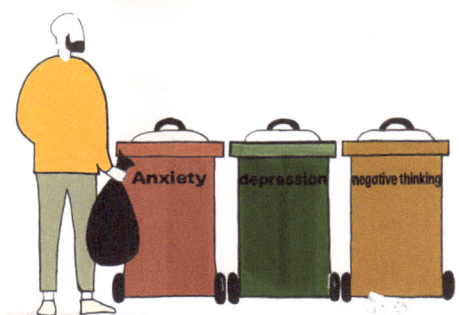

For example: The purpose of a car is for transportation, but we can observe that at least a gas engine car produces exhaust. The purpose of the gas engine is to produce power to drive the car, but the engine also produces exhaust—as a by-product—that is excreted into the environment. The product is the engine, its purpose is to power the car.

Exhaust is a by-product. One could say it serves no purpose, but still must be reckoned with.

Similarly, if we were to imagine an automobile factory, we could say the factory's true purpose was to produce cars. But if we looked at the factory from the outside, we would observe that it also produces smoke. Yes, the factory also produces smoke, but the smoke is a by-product of its true purpose of production. Now imagine for a moment if the smoke coming out of the stacks was re-circulated back into the factory, just how impossible it would become for the car assemblers to do their jobs because they would be choking on the smoke.

Now we can apply these concepts to our mental lives. The **purpose of our brain is for our survival,** and our brain produce many wonderful things that aid our survival. But we can also notice that our brain also produces many things that actually get in the way of our survival. In mindfulness, I call these negative co-productions by-products or mental waste.

As human beings, we are unique in being able to be aware of our inner mental life, but much of what we are aware is rather disturbing and not useful.

Mindfulness teachings suggest that all of these disturbing and non-useful mental productions are tantamount to mental waste material, just like the exhaust from a car and the smoke from an automobile factory.

And, the fundamental challenge to all humans, unlike with our physical waste, **there is no built-in or adequate mental excretion mechanism for this mental waste.** This then leads us to the realization of just how essential it is for our survival and well-being to develop a tool to help us **problem solve how to eliminate this mental waste**. The tool I have developed to accomplish this, I call **mental dialysis.**

Unlike kidney dialysis, we can't use an artificial machine to remove toxic mental waste. But we do need to develop and learn how to utilize our prefrontal cortex, which, like a **Swiss Army Knife,** contains the blades of realizations, selectivity, and the shifting of attention to facilitate the removal of this mental waste.

Mindfulness training teaches us to be aware of our built-in mental Swiss Army Knife and to learn how to utilize all of its blades to our advantage. Like a hunter using their knife to carve out the best and greatest number of meat portions, or the butcher in the grocery market using the knife to trim the fat to make what we eat healthier, we can learn to use the carving blade of our prefrontal cortex to help us carve through our noxious experiences—so many of which are indigestible or even bad for our health.

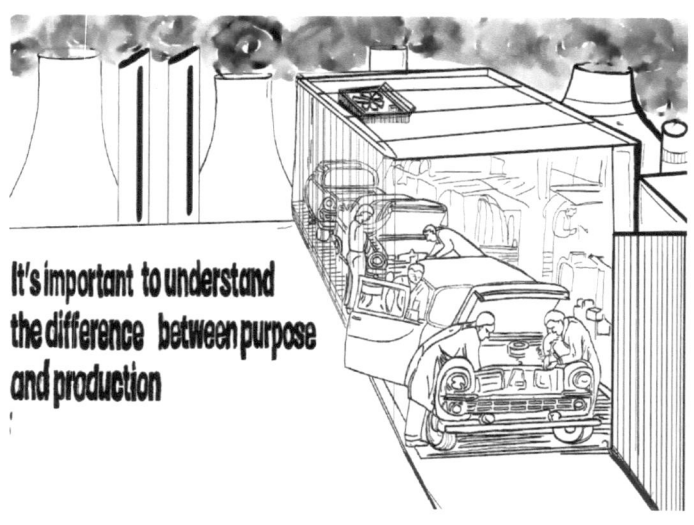

Negative Thinking

Why do humans think so negatively about themselves?
What can we do about this?

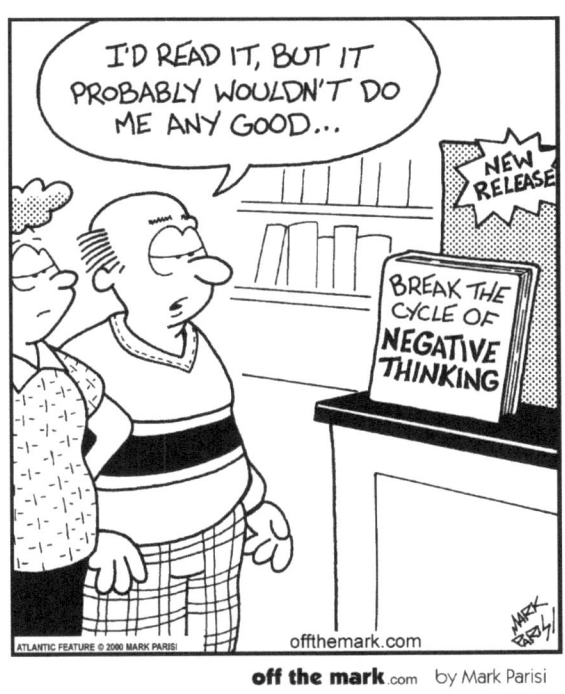

It has long been thought that humans are unique because we can think. Apart from new evidence that indicates as least some elementary forms of cognition do exist in animals which allows them some ability to solve problems and plan ahead; what is unique about human thought is certainly not that most of what we think is useless. Nor is it that a significant portion is actually harmful. It seems our uniqueness as human beings lies less in the fact that we can think, but in our ability to think and reflect about what we are thinking—that is in our ability to meta-think.

Our capacity to meta-think comes from our prefrontal cortex, and mindfulness training can be seen as specific learning exercises designed to help us evolve and improve our capacity to meta-think, to reflect on our thoughts, feelings, and impulses with greater clarity, and to realize we can—and often have to—make better choices as to which thoughts, feelings, and impulses to attend to.

Our advantage as human beings is firstly because we have the most highly developed prefrontal cortex—we have the capacity, the horsepower built-in. Secondly, that this capacity is open for development, and can be strengthened through education and training.

In mindfulness training, we train ourselves to separate our useful, beneficial, problem solving, creative and inspired thoughts from the counterproductive, nearsighted, rationalizing—and way too often—ridiculous and outright harmful ones.

We can also learn to be more selective about our feelings, as it seems we would be much better off if we learned to select the feelings of love, compassion and joy over feelings of shame, resentment and vindictiveness. We might consider this 'mental selection feature' as a special feature that allows our us to make more enlightened choices and 'selections' today and tomorrow, in our present lifetime, not based on genetic mutations that require generations of time-consuming extinctions before new and improved models are introduced eons later.

It seems this **mental selection feature** was selected by natural selection to give us a huge survival advantage. Most of us are unaware we have this feature or how to utilize it. Mindfulness training teaches us to develop our prefrontal cortex's ability to operate like a jukebox and only select the songs that truly brings music to our ears and to turn off (or at least turn down) the noisy recordings. We can use our own intelligence and awareness to distinguish our best and most adaptive features of our brains and cultivate and develop those; while minimizing our worst features before they get us into any greater trouble.

The **mindfulness homework** that all members of my mindfulness groups do each week to train their meta-thinking capacity is to keep a weekly diary of their thoughts and feelings: recognizing, distinguishing and separating their negative counterproductive thoughts, feelings and impulses that come from their LOWER SELF, (AMYGDALA), from the higher level of thoughts and feelings generated in that special evolved area of our brain: HIGHER SELF (PREFRONTAL CORTEX).

This mental exercise is to help provide us with a mental filtration mechanism—an artificial mental kidney, so to speak—that allows us to identify, but not dwell on, negative and toxic thoughts, feelings, or impulses.

We learn to hold the awareness of what is toxic within our mental fork in our left hand, and then use our mental knife in our right hand to be selective, PAYING ATTENTION to, and SHIFTING OUR ATTENTION to what we are about to put in our mouths, exercising a moment of quality control to ensure that it is safe, edible, and beneficial. This is the same kind of sorting mechanism we use when we separate our important mail from our junk mail.

Typically, we glance at our junk mail for a nanosecond, just enough time to recognize what it is before quickly throwing it in the trash so to keep our physical space uncluttered.

In my mindfulness groups I bring a waste basket into the group room that has the sign on it "mental waste" as a reminder that we do need to also throw out our negative thoughts, our anxiety, self-doubts and recriminations, and our resentments, as well as our paper cups and straws.

I often have them write down their toxic thoughts and feelings on scraps of paper and instruct them to then crumple them up and actually throw them into the waste basket so that they learn to take this exercise: litter-ally!

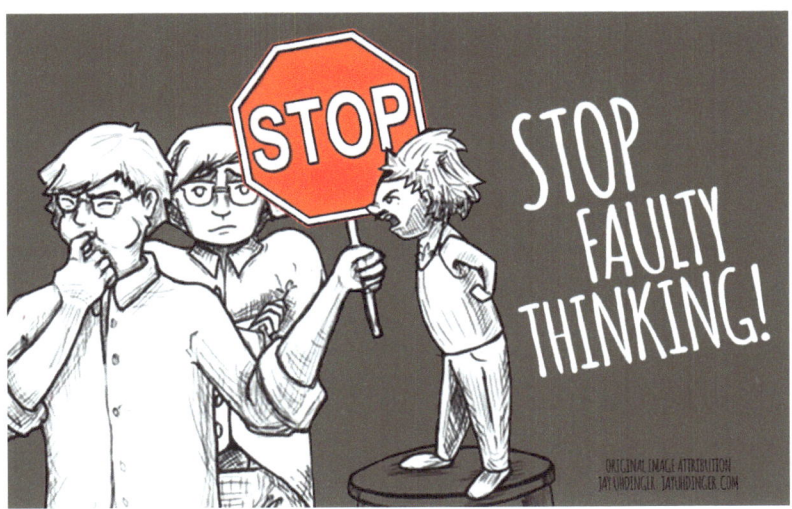

Environmental awareness has also now trained us to further separate the plastics, from the paper, from the electronics. But we need to become comparably more sophisticated in identifying and separating out the various kinds of mental trash we carry.

We learn to do this mental filtration exercise with determination, because we realize that there is no built-in mechanism for the elimination of MENTAL WASTE, and we realize if we don't problem-solve some way of removing this mental waste from our minds, we will suffer mentally. Without a means of removal, the mental waste just accumulates. It is no wonder we feel lousy so often.

The pictures of the amount of plastic waste dumped into our oceans are daunting but a reminder of how important it is to not allow our brain to become a dumping and burial ground for our noxious experiences. While the plastic may be out of view, it is harming the ocean and is choking the life inside it.

Our prefrontal cortex is the brain module that gives of the capacity to realize these pollution problems not only in the ocean atmosphere and in our minds, but also the capacity to problem-solve and develop a strategy to figure out what to do about it.

Our prefrontal cortex is our driver, our overseer, our selector-in-chief, enabling us to go to the store to pick the food we will eat, the clothes we wear, the cars we buy, and the books we read. It reminds us to brush our teeth and to dental floss, take our medicines, see the doctor, spend time with our children, connect with friends and family, work hard and pay our bills, take out the trash, and ask for help when needed.

It is our realizer-in-chief, and realizes **we also need to take out our mental trash, and not be a receptacle for other people's mental trash.** We understand that if our kidneys have failed and we can't free our bodies of the toxin BUN (blood urea nitrogen), we will suffer, if not die, and must turn to renal dialysis (an artificial kidney) to remove it. **So too, we realize since we are not born with any built-in, mental waste excretion mechanism, no mental kidney, so to speak, we must create one for ourselves**. We understand that mindfulness training is the device we can develop that allows us to be aware of, identify, and remove, this toxic mental waste.

Mindfulness training calls upon us to do these mental filtration exercises because we understand better that we are capable of, and need to access, our mental

Negative Thinking

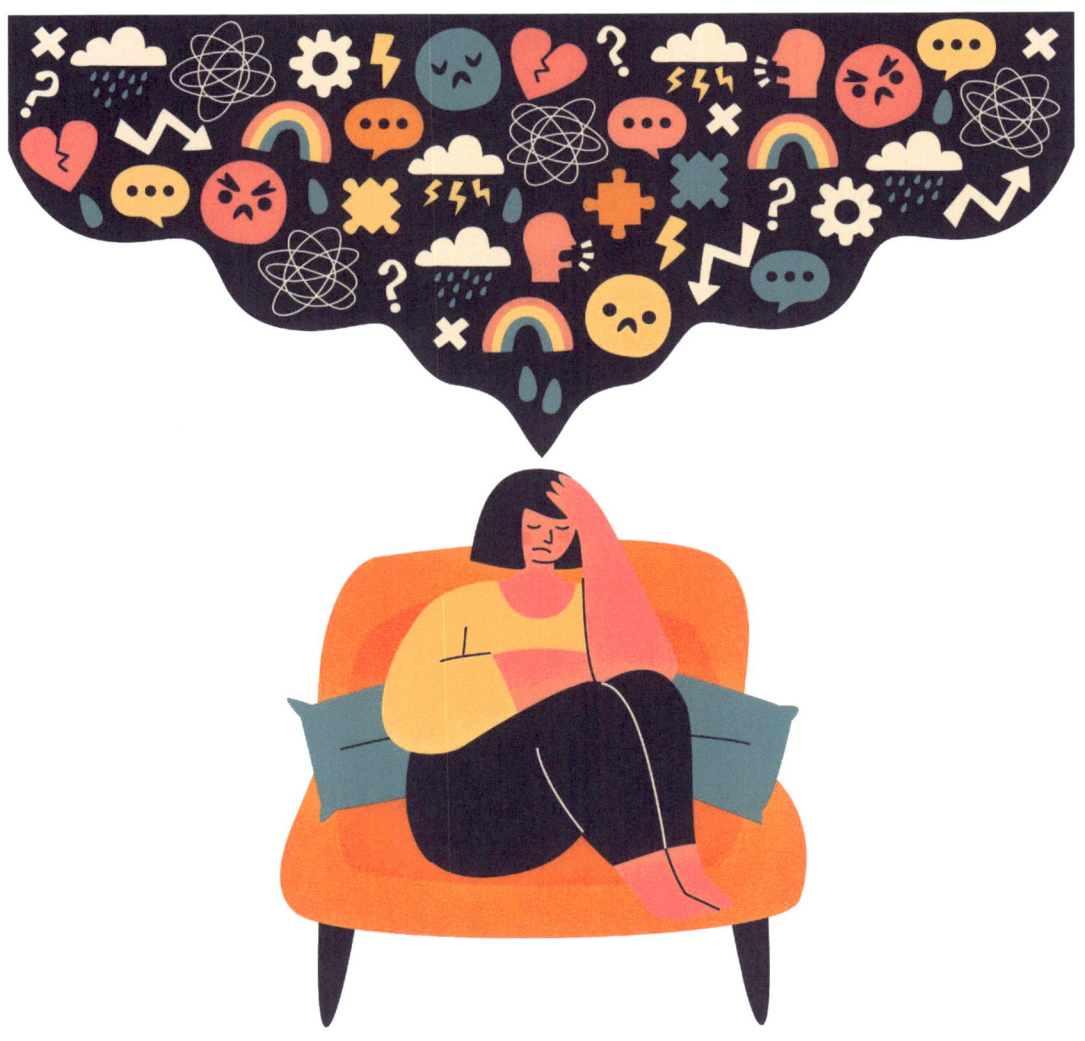

oxygen-like thoughts, feelings, and impulses that nourish us and help us to feel alive and to thrive. We also quarantine our mental carbon dioxide-like, thoughts, feelings and impulses, which interfere with our well-being and which we need to learn to catch and release. Imagine for a moment what would happen to the automobile workers if the smoke from the factory—instead of being released into the atmosphere—stayed in the factory. Productivity would grind to a halt.

Unless and until we learn to remove our mental waste, our full potential as human beings will be seriously impaired. Put more positively, just think of what we may be capable of—our upside potential—when we learn to remove this mental muck!

Meta-Thinking

Meta-thinking or thinking about our thinking (and thinking about our feelings) gives us the opportunity to not get hijacked by a thought or feeling, but to first be aware of each thought or feeling. Then by thinking about it, to carefully examine each one to assess its quality and usefulness. We become ad hoc jewelry appraisers putting the magnifying glass to our eye to inspect for the quality of the thought and feeling before concluding its value and buying it.

We learn through this exercise to **become a witness to and appraiser of our thoughts and feelings**. When we do, we realize that most of what we think, and feel is far removed from being real diamonds. Yet, we also want to be ready when the few true diamonds of our thinking come along. A good fisherman learns to recognize the tug of a really big fish, and even if their mind wandered off, will quickly shift gears to reel it in.

This capacity for alertness to whatever arises is an essential part of mindfulness training. Learning to reel in the tugs of love, compassion, kindness, gratitude, and positive thoughts of self-worth and hopefulness, and avoid the tugs of bitterness, resentment, self-hatred, shame and despair, is crucial to our well-being.

Our mental capacities for alertness, awareness, **becoming a non-judgmental witness to our mental activity**, and carefully appraising and selecting the best of our mental litter are all derived from our prefrontal cortex. With mindfulness training, we develop our ability to make these distinctions between higher and lower level thoughts. Higher level thoughts are purposeful, beneficial, and useful, while lower level thoughts are counter-productive and often outright harmful.

Our prefrontal cortex is the part of our brain that not only makes these distinctions, but also **understands why making these distinctions is so important**.

Our brainstem neurons can recognize the difference between high and low levels of glucose and make automatic adjustments accordingly, but have no capacity to understand why these distinctions and adjustments are so important. Lower levels of brain functioning operate in an automatic, "Just do it" manner, while our higher levels function with the realization of what and why it needs to be done, and can purposely direct its energies accordingly. If the automaticity is beneficial to us and our oxygen level is adjusted upwards or downward, we benefit. However, if our body's automatic response is over the top—like when our ankles swell excessively when injured—we suffer more pain than is helpful and we have to ice the swelling to compensate. Mindfulness training teaches us to become aware of our intensity and frequency of our automatic negative thoughts and feelings. We learn to cool off and ice our negative thoughts, feelings, and impulses, so to speak.

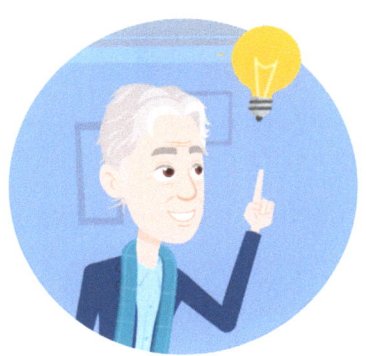

Selectivity is key. A baker knows how important it is to separate the whites from the yolks. A baker also understands that these distinctions and separations require attention and care, and that doing so results in a higher-quality baked product. Our cells that line our lungs are specialized in making careful distinctions between oxygen and carbon dioxide, but have no clue why they do so.

A core mindfulness teaching is that we can train our prefrontal cortex neurons to make comparably essential mental distinctions between those thoughts and feelings that are like our mental oxygen and help us to feel well and glad to be alive. Those thoughts and feelings that are deleterious, and affect us like mental carbon dioxide, we need to find some way to release and exhale.

An essential teaching of mindfulness is that much of what we think and feel actually makes us not feel well. Mindfulness training teaches how to be aware of this mental muck and how to liberate ourselves from it. A jeweler knows that it's not the quick first glance that determines a jewel's value, but rather the second third slower and more careful, focused observations which get a more accurate and useful assessment.

Mindfulness training allows us to look at our thoughts, feeling and impulses with the same kind of care, attention and quality of assessment. We develop an ever-emerging trained eye, separate out, and utilize the healthier whites, so that the higher cholesterol yolk of our lower brain no longer controls us.

One of the exercises I have developed for mindfulness training to facilitate this selection process is what I call **mental skeet shooting.** In skeet shooting, clay discs are launched into the air while a person with a rifle aims, shoots, and fires at them with the intention of hitting them and knocking them out of the air.

In mental skeet shooting, we become aware that our insignificant and often counter-productive thoughts, feelings, and impulses are being launched all the time. Our prefrontal cortex is our rifle. It is loaded with the bullets of awareness and has the ability to aim, focus, fire, and watch our mental clay discs—our thoughts—fall to the ground. With practice, we can become really good at recognizing and shooting down our negative and counter-productive thoughts, always remembering that **we are the shooter and not what we are shooting at.**

With our meta-thinking we can begin to pause, reflect, become more aware of, and become curious about our self-harming impulses. We learn that these are built-in to the lower human psyche of all human beings. In order to understand why our brain contains this module of self-harming negativity, we need to learn about the amygdala and how our amygdala is similar to and different from that of other living creatures.

The amygdala (the fight or flight area of the brain) is a very a small part of our primitive brain which is devoted to help generate behaviors to increase our chances of survival in the wild.

Our brain needed to generate enough offensive aggression to pursue and even kill sources of food in order to avoid starvation. Defensive aggression was necessary to protect ourselves from predators pursuing us for their meal. Accompanying these feelings of fear and aggression were the emergence of their primitive cognitive counterparts.

When we were fearful, we were more likely to think suspiciously and with paranoia, that something might be out there trying to get us. When we were starving and on the prowl for food, we were more likely to think others might be on the prowl after us as well. We can see that this hodgepodge of hunger, fear of starvation, fear of being eaten or maimed, automatic spewing of the offensive and defensive aggression, and its accompanying suspicious, paranoid and projective primitive thinking, might keep us anxious and on edge most of the day and night.

Despite the discomfort they caused, they might, in the end, have actually kept us alive. **Natural selection chose survival over quality of life**. Mindfulness training teaches us that this dis-ease is built into our brain. But **natural selection** also incorporated into our brain the **capacity to learn to transcend our lower wiring** when our survival instincts might become counter-productive or even harmful.

It seems our amygdala was much more useful to us back in the day. In today's modern world, we have switches to turn on and off most of what we need and don't need. We turn the heat on when we need it, and off when we don't. We turn on the AC when we need it, and off when we don't. However, **there is no on-off switch for our amygdala**. It runs like the refrigerator, always on and always consuming our attention and energy while no longer providing the same beneficial function for which it was designed.

When we compare our brain with other brains, **we realize we indeed have the best brain on the evolutionary market!** However, when we compare our amygdala with the amygdala of other species, we realize the human amygdala has many shortcomings. One day, in one of the mindfulness groups I run, a fly joined the group gathering and kept landing and taking off from one group member to the next. In a manner of minutes, distressed group members, increasingly annoyed by the fly, took hard swats at the fly without quite realizing they were actually hitting themselves. In addition, they started to feel and think negative thoughts about themselves for not being able to get the little bugger. I paused the group, and shifted their attention to the wonderful mindfulness teaching moment we had just stumbled upon: an opportunity to observe and learn the difference between the fly's amygdala (its fight or flight module) and ours.

At its core, the fly's escape module successfully allowed the fly to escape the repeated swats even though its brain was smaller than the size of a pea. Meanwhile, our human amygdala directed it owners to both be aggressive toward the fly AND toward itself: swatting itself and saying derogatory things to itself about not being able to kill it.

This **self-directed negativity is unique to human beings**. Mindfulness training teaches us to become aware of this self-directed negativity and learn not to personalize it.

Since it is hard-wired into our brain, every human being struggles with it. Mindfulness training then teaches us how to unhook ourselves from the barbed wire of this self-directed negativity before we hurt ourselves or others.

At another mental health center where I work, one of the psychiatric nurses I work with was called out on Christmas Eve day because her husband, a UPS deliverer, was bitten by a dog delivering a package. The dog's aggressive, territorial behavior was its amygdala in action. The dog had no mental capacity to realize that the deliverer was not an intruder or to consider that what was being delivered might be a dog bone for its Christmas present!

But a dog's aggression is directed outwardly and never against itself. If you throw a dog a Frisbee and it doesn't catch it, it never thinks: 'What a spaz!' The dog just eagerly signals to throw it again and again. It seems that dogs just want to have fun! Moreover, it seems they know how to have fun as they are spared the human amygdala's capacity for self-recrimination and seem to be much happier because of it.

Mindfulness training helps us become aware of just how important it is that we learn how to override this small, yet potent brain module that served us better in the past than the present. We also learn that one of the psychological ways that the amygdala dominates us is by how handcuffed our identity—our sense of who we are—has become unwittingly linked to this small and rather obsolete area of our brain.

Mindfulness training then also helps us to purposely redirect our attention and psychic energies away from this more primitive relic to our prefrontal cortex—our best and vastly under-utilized part of our brain—which has so many more useful capabilities. Our prefrontal cortex which generates our meta-thinking provides the keys to unhook us from our lower level thoughts and feelings, and to unlock us from the many psychological ways we have become handcuffed to our amygdala.

The Evolution of the Human Minds(s)

We can understand ourselves better when we understand how the human brain works. We can then understand the human brain better if we understand how our brain is similar to, and different from, other brains. All evolution strives to give its owner distinct advantages in its struggle for survival. Our species survived and thrived not by being faster, bigger, or stronger, but by adding cognitive, emotional, and linguistic capacities allowing us to think, speak, write, remember, imagine, comprehend, reason, plan, problem-solve, and understand abstract binary concepts like time and space, illness and wellness.

We can intelligently reason about cause and effect, make higher-level distinctions between what is alive and dead, animate and inanimate, friend and foe, real and imagined, true and untrue, authentic and phony, or beneficial and harmful.

Our prefrontal cortex allows us to imagine—to see in our minds the way things look from others' perspectives—which in turn leads us to the higher emotions of compassion and empathy. Because of our enhanced prefrontal cortex , we can focus our mental attention in ways analogous to a cat stalking a mouse—but for higher purposes than the next meal—that allows us to study, learn, master, love, care and protect at levels never seen before. We then also can appreciate beauty, know right from wrong, understand fairness and justice, enjoy and create music, and feel joyful bliss.

Our prefrontal cortex allows us to imagine what we might do (rehearse) before actually doing it, giving us the opportunity to either upgrade what we had in mind, nip it in the bud, censor it, or modify it.

Human beings understand that living organisms don't live forever—which allows us, in turn, to more fully celebrate being alive. Our brain's uniqueness goes beyond the extension of previous specious capabilities, moving toward the development of brand-new capabilities.

Our human brain allows us the unique advantage of being aware of our internal mental life, which in turn allows us to be aware of both our positive and negative

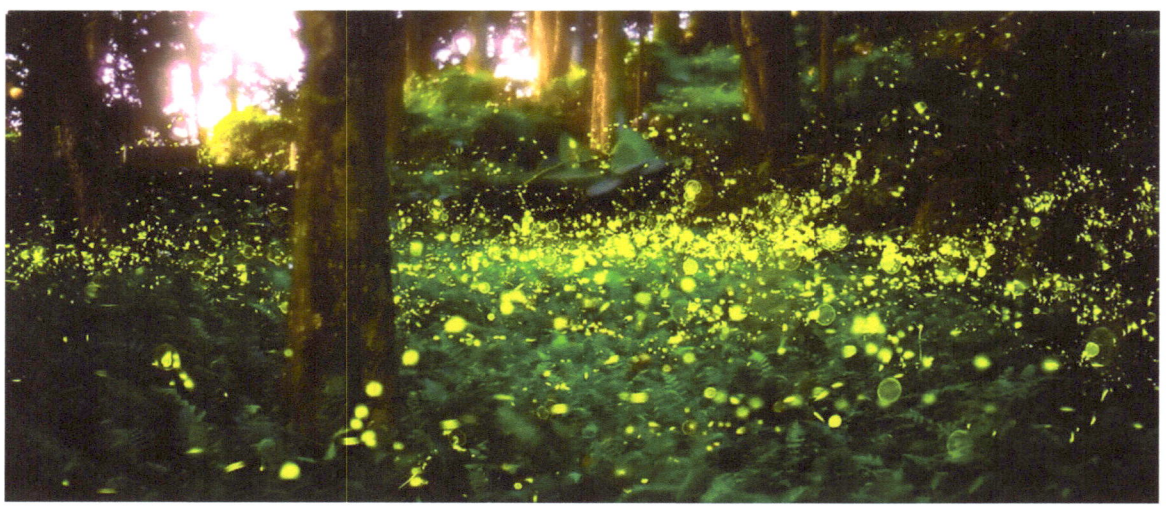

internal mental assets. This inner mental awareness then allows us to learn to distinguish and strengthen our internal positive mental capabilities while curtailing the disadvantageous ones.

Our higher-level cognitive abilities include our ability to analyze, select, reflect, learn, comprehend, understand abstract ideas, metaphors, and analogies, teach, communicate by language, music and art, to visualize mentally, and to anticipate and predict results. Higher cognition emerged from the building blocks of lower cognition.

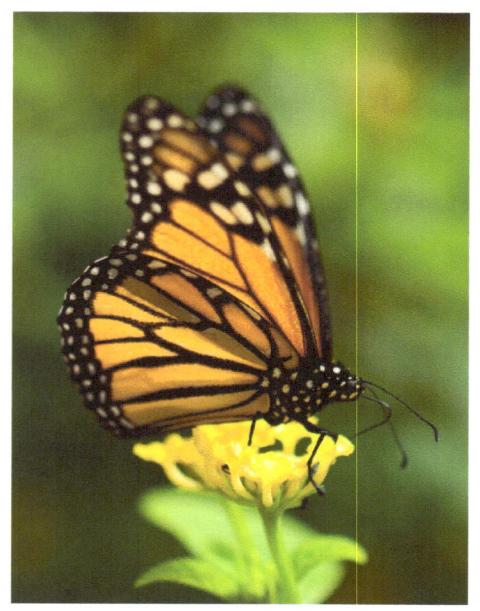

One of the essential tasks of mindfulness training is to help us become aware of and distinguish between our higher and lower cognitions, as well as our higher and lower emotions. One of the essential tenants of mindfulness training is that we have overvalued thinking altogether.

I remember taking my first philosophy course in college and being mesmerized by Descartes' famous dictum "Cogito ergo sum", "I think therefore I am." It wasn't until sometime after graduating medical school that I wondered

The Evolution of the Human Mind(s)

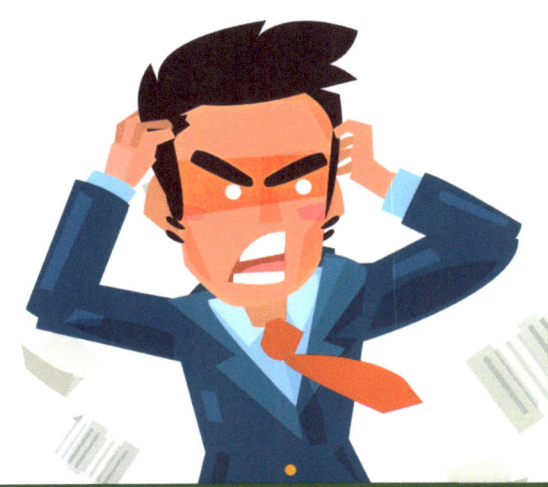

I lower level think therefore I suffer!

I think therefore I am

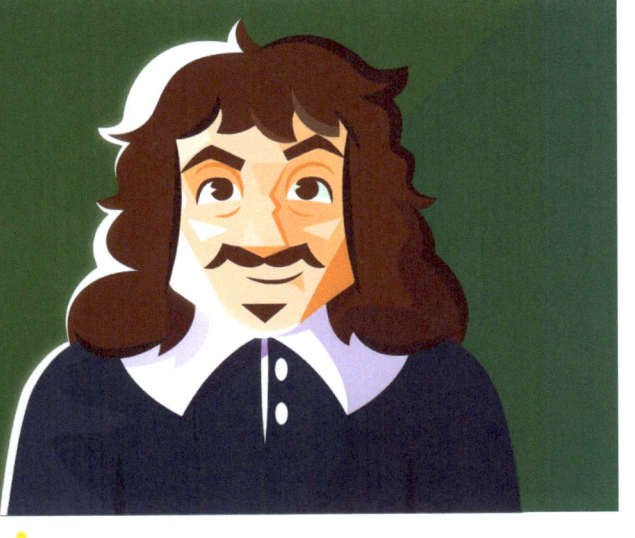

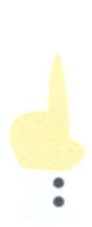
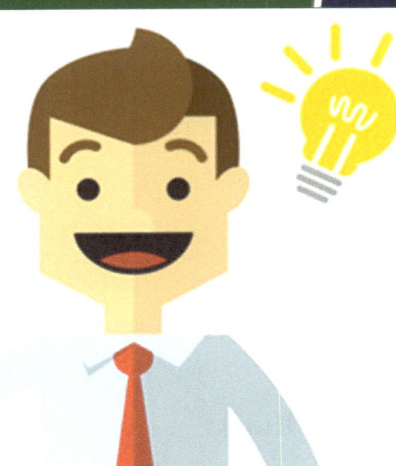

I higher level or meta-think therefore I am happy!

why it wasn't "I breathe therefore I am."

It occurred to me that most of our thoughts are rather insubstantial. In the words of Perry Mason, most of our thoughts are effectively "irrelevant and immaterial!"

Mindfulness training teaches that thoughts are like mental fireflies—quick flashes, that soon disappear. We are encouraged to observe them, but not to chase or collect them. One of the benefits we derive by becoming a witness to our thoughts is that we realize that very few of our thoughts are like butterflies: both worth the chase and the catch.

Entwined with our lower level thoughts is our lower levels of reasoning like being suspicious, rationalizing, justifying, blaming, jumping to conclusions, and being judgmental. Mythologies developed in ancient Greece and Egypt to explain cause and effect. The lower-level reasoning explained, for example, why the crops did not grow in a particular season.

They 'thought' that Zeus must have been having a fight with Hera. While this thinking was creative and now entertaining, this "thinking" actually compelled the populace to behave in a way, making some rather gruesome sacrifices, so as to appease these imagined gods. Not that long ago we thought and believed the earth was the center of the universe.

Today, we are bombarded by conspiracy theories, politically motivated explanations strikingly devoid of substantiating facts. Part of the work in alcohol and substance treatment is uncovering the myths that users have developed about both their drugs and about themselves. It is rather humbling to become aware of just how many idiotic thoughts we do have.

Mindfulness trains us to spot our idiotic thoughts quickly so that we are not led around in counter-productive circles by them. When a person who has been 15 years sober from drinking has the seeming benign thought: 'I should by now be able to have just one,' a Mindfulness training five-alarm siren goes off to warn its owner of the danger of that thought.

A person who has a peanut allergy never thinks "I should be able to have just one", without the image of their airway closing up popping up to help them quickly let go of the peanut's allure. **They understand and accept the life-threatening nature of the peanut allergy, and quickly move on to thinking about what they can eat safely.**

Mindfulness training not only helps us be more aware of the harmfulness of the substances we might use, but also **the harmfulness of the very thinking which steers us in the direction of those substances in the first place.**

We can see that our prefrontal cortex evolved to become our largest lobe and brain module to perform these kinds of higher-order executive functions, such as spotting those thoughts that would put ourselves in harm's way and nip them in the bud.

But what are these impulses to self-harm doing in the human psyche in the first place?

In 400 BC Hippocrates said: "From our brain alone arises **our pleasures, joy, laughter and sorrow just as well as our sorrows, pains, grief and tears." To this insight I would add that from our brain alone also arises our impulsivity, sensitivity to rejection, anger, rage, impatience, judgmental tendencies, self-hatred, jealousy, guilt, shame, impaired sense of worth, boredom, depression, anxiety, moodiness, and impulses to self-harm and self-sabotage!**

To further understand true self-destructiveness, we need to **distinguish intended from unintended self-harm**. In a rather amazing segment from the documentary *Our Planet* narrated by David Attenborough on Netflix, a group of animal-loving naturalists were shown filming from a distance a group of walruses who had climbed on land for a brief rest and snooze only to find the beach too rocky to rest. They shimmied up to higher ground to find a more comfortable resting spot and napped there. When they were awakened by their hunger for fish and desire to get back to the ocean, they began to shimmy down only to discover their weight going downhill led them to topple down the rocky incline, one after another and suffer severe injuries or die.

The naturalists who were filming this could only watch in horror. The naturalists because of their human brain could comprehend what the walrus brain could not comprehend; the 'gravity' of the situation.

Now we must ask ourselves as treatment providers, friends, and family members: "What is it that alcohol and substance users fail to comprehend about the gravity of their usage even though they possess the human brain fully capable of comprehending it?" The general explanation substance users give these days is that, 'I do it because I am an addict', hides more than it reveals, and reflects the kind of lower-level reasoning discussed earlier. **We need to get at the psychological root of our self-injuriousness** here as our advanced, ever-capable human brain nonetheless also possesses a module that, left unchecked, propels us to self-harm and use substances without any true regard for their consequences.

Our brain equips us with modules that are in direct conflict. One module operates like a gas pedal; the other like a brake. The gas pedal generates the impulses to use, and to actively disregard the potential horrible consequences. Our brake tells us this is a very bad idea. Mindfulness introduces the term **"Duel" Diagnosis** to describe this epic human, never ending battle between our higher impulses (the brake) to self-care and self-protect, and the lower impulses (the gas pedal) to use without regard to consequences.

Braking (keeping ourselves from self-harming) is one of the essential ways we act to self-care and self-protect. Our braking capability is derived from out prefrontal cortex and the impulse to self-harm and self-neglect is derived from the amygdala.

When we look at alcohol and substance use struggles through the lenses of self-injury impulses, and compare ourselves to the plight of the walrus herd, our impulse to jump off a cliff, or stop at the package store, for the fun and pleasure of it, is simply reckless. The walrus instinct impulse and survival instinct to get back to the water while it backfired was healthy, in that its aim and purpose was for survival. Like the walrus, we too have comprehension failures. But unlike the walrus we do have the capacity to comprehend, and even to comprehend our comprehension problems.

We are called upon to understand the unique mystery of why one area of our brain propels us to use while another area knows that it is because of our use that we will likely lose our marriage, kids, and jobs, in addition to suffering from pancreatitis, liver failure, or even death, yet we do it anyway!

The Evolution of the Human Mind(s)

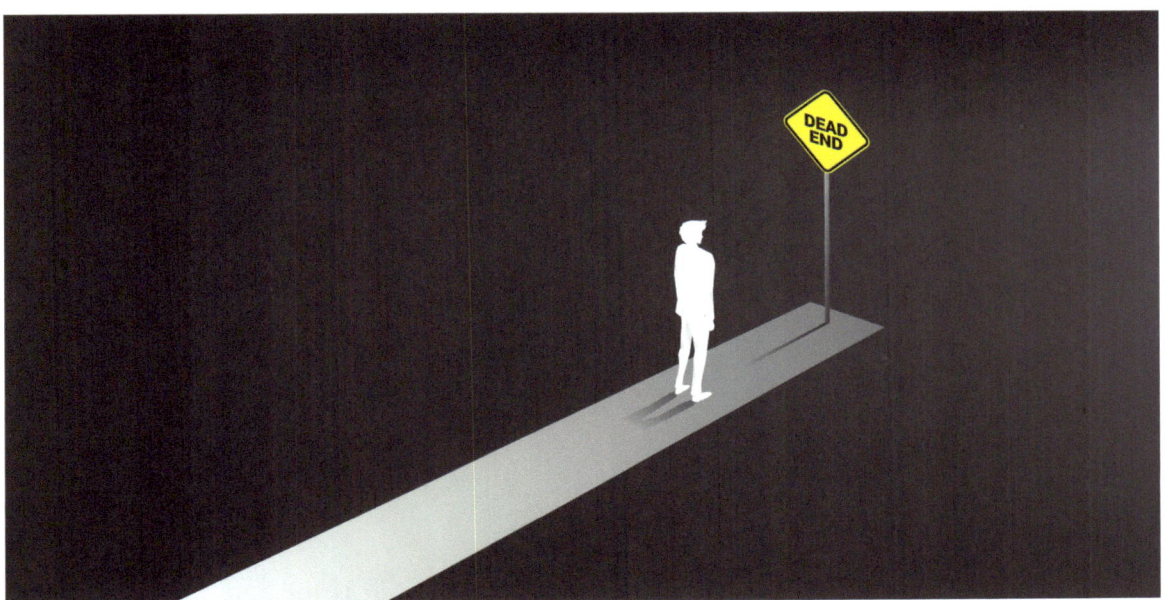

Most people have never wondered **why human beings are the only living entity that has ever existed that self-injures** in this "I know better but do it anyway," fashion. In mindfulness we tackle this question straight on: If we are to understand the brain as an organ of survival, how can we also understand it generating impulses to self-harm and self-injure with tragically staggering numbers of lethal consequences? Substance users tend to mythologize and romanticize the substances they use: "It's the only thing that works for me; it's my drug of choice!" At the same time, they have an uncanny ability to downplay or even outright deny the self-destructiveness of their usage and the inevitable harm that will follow. We must remember, these are fellow humans equipped with an ever-capable human brain and are not like the walrus returning to the ocean when they shimmy on down to the pusher, the pub, or the package store.

The dual and dueling model of the brain that I introduce in Mindfulness helps us begin to comprehend better what we are up against. Our upper brain and our upper mind readily pursue one set of goals, while the lower brain and its attendant lower mind is driven in the pursuit of different and lesser goals. The **lower brain is modulated by immediate reward or the anticipation of immediate reward.** This **reward system** is modulated by **dopamine**—a **neurotransmitter** found in large quantities in

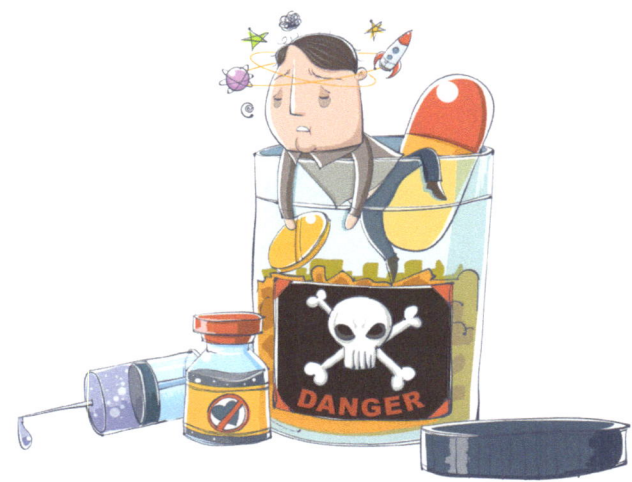

an area of the brain called the **nucleus accumbens** which is located, you guessed it, adjacent to our nemesis, our amygdala.

The goal of this part of the brain is simply to propel us to get as much pleasure as possible, as quickly as possible. It is this very small area of our lower brain that craves and obsesses about substances that will activate dopamine. Even just imagining obtaining the dopamine-triggering substances begins the cascade of dopamine release. The amygdala, nucleus accumbens, and hippocampus (traumatic memory center) are all next-door neighbors in a small area of our brain and function together like Boston's old combat zone that was **not a safe place to walk by day and was even worse at night.**

What most people do not understand is that **dopamine is a chemical form of Fool's Gold**. It is not what it is 'cracked' up to be and is far from the 'best high' we are capable of experiencing. People chase dopamine highs as if they are the Holy Grail worthy of sacrificing one's life. In fact, **dopamine is a cheap, short-lived high that comes at the enormous price tag of addiction**, self and other injury, unnecessary family and marital break-up, and decimated careers, taking an immeasurable adverse impact on our kids, nevermind our brain, pancreas, liver and self-esteem. Nicotine is a substance that stimulates dopamine. Most smokers are unaware that nicotine is a substance naturally produced in the tobacco leaf that is a **NEUROTOXIN.** It is produced to protect the tobacco leaf from insects that would chew its leaves by **poisoning the nerve cells of the insects.** When we remember that our basic nerve cells are so similar to even those in insects, we can begin to more fully appreciate how the pleasurable effects of smoking are only fooling us into self-harm.

What we also have not fully realized is that **we have other neurotransmitters that are worth the chase**: endorphins, enkephalins, anandamide, and oxytocin are fabulous neurotransmitters located primarily in the prefrontal cortex that allow us true contentment, true and lasting satisfaction, inner peace, and joy, and they can be accessed naturally and have NO SIDE EFFECTS!

Chasing dopamine is so misguided. It is like the becoming obsessed with the pursuit of a prostitute or a one-night stand knowing the next morning when you wake up from your revelry, you will be quite worried you may have contracted an STD. Driving this misguided pursuit may be loneliness, and our insecurities may be about our ability to find a more meaningful, lasting and viable connection.

The other morning, I was listening to some incredible music by Miles Davis and was imagining my **endorphins dancing like sugar plums**, when my memory flashed on the old Camel cigarette advertisement: 'I'd walk a mile for a Camel!' And then the thought that popped into my mind was, **"I'd ride an uncomfortable camel just to hear Miles!**'

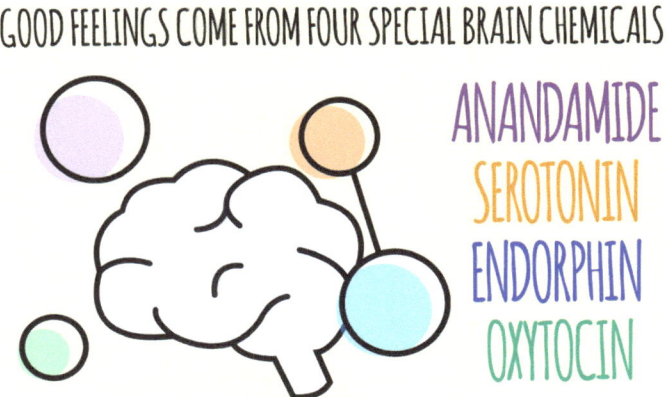

The issue here is to recognize the extreme risks we will take for an immediate reward with rather dire longer-term consequences. We could make a different choice—which may be inconvenient in the moment, but it would lead to a truly satisfying and lasting long-term result without any risk.

Mindfulness helps to guide us away from the impulsivity that so easily leads us to step into potholes. It also helps us to become more focused on the pursuit of what we truly want and need, knowing that, if we were just to pause to stop and think about it more constructively, **we don't truly want something that will bring unwanted consequences into our lives.**

One of the advantages of our prefrontal cortex that allows us to study and learn about our own brain is that we can **realize we have been wasting our time chasing the wrong neurotransmitter**. Just as many Covid-19 vaccine pursuits will be dropped once a really effective vaccine is discovered, mindfulness training teaches us to shift our energies to the endorphin, enkephalin, anandamide, and oxytocin-releasing activities of physical exercise, study and learning, meaningful and lasting connections, skill development, hobby pursuits, and all that develops our ability to connect with life, develop our love and compassion and be of benefit to others, and away from the dopamine sought short-lived and often misleading pleasures that come at such a huge cost.

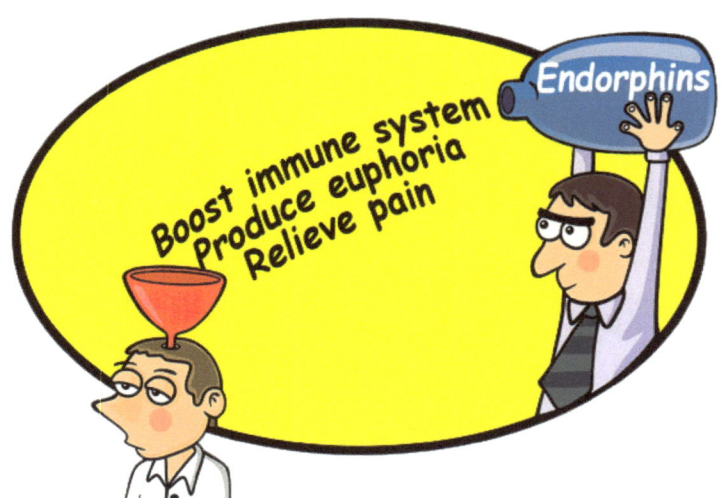

The Role of Trauma

Space does not allow me to go into this issue in great detail in this writing, but I would truly be remiss if I did not include it, as there is a rather **high correlation between PTSD and substance use**. Moreover, mindfulness training offers a lot to consider in the treatment of PTSD.

People often turn to using substances to cope with the memories of traumatic pasts including mental, physical, and sexual abuse. Often the substance is used to numb the feelings associated with the memories of these traumatic experiences, which often continue to haunt throughout one's life. Learning about the brain helps us to better put these awful experiences into a better and more useful perspective.

Firstly, we begin to understand that **the perpetrators of our trauma have or had an amygdala also,** and it was their failure to learn how to manage and more effectively regulate their amygdala that generated their untoward conduct. The purpose of understanding this is not to let them off the hook for what they did, but to further motivate us to focus on accomplishing for ourselves what they failed to accomplish for themselves: the effective management of our own amygdala.

Brain anatomy shows us that traumatic memories are stored in the hippocampus (another small area of our brain that is adjacent to the amygdala). **The hippocampus records and stores traumatic memories, and then throughout our lives, tortures us further by playing the memories back, over and over again**.

What happened to us should never have happened in the first place, never mind repeatedly by remembering through our adult lives.. Neuroscience can now document that both what we imagine and remember can have almost the same devastating effect as the actual experience itself. Feelings of anger, hurt, resentment and bitterness that are activated each time we remember only strengthens our amygdala.

Mindfulness training teaches us we must learn to weaken amygdala activity, and to do so **we need to shift our attention away from traumatic memories**—not to pretend they didn't happen, but to actively lessen their hold on us. While these traumatic memories are made with sticky glue, we need to learn to let them go. As they try to hold onto us, we must learn to not to let them hold us back.

One gentleman I saw who endured unspeakable violence in his childhood reported to me he could not remember a single positive memory from his childhood. I told him that despite the horrors he had experienced, there were positive memories stored in is brain as well, and I suggested he search for them.

The next week he reported that for the first time, he remembered riding his bicycle as a kid. Mindfulness training teaches us not to allow the traumatic memories to bully away the positive memories we are entitled to.

As kids, we were at the mercy of the abuse and neglect of our caretakers in ways that were quite detrimental to our well being.

However, **it is essential we learn not to pick up today where our caretakers left off yesterday**. If they denigrated us, we must learn to stop denigrating ourselves. If they did not care for us well or protect us from harm, we have to learn to take especially good care of ourselves now.

It is essential we realize that when we use alcohol and drugs now, it is we who have become the perpetrators today—and our bodies and self-worth are the victims. There was little we could have done about our childhood situations; there is much we can do about our adult lives.

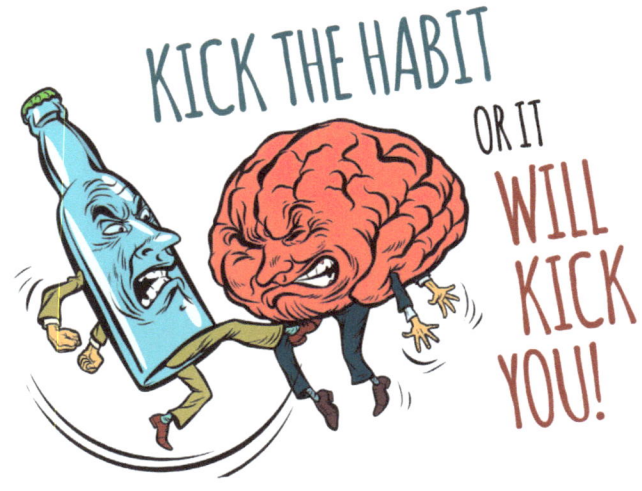

Role of Medication

Mindfulness training offers some important guidelines regarding using medication in the treatment of alcohol and substance use disorders.

1. Firstly, it makes a **fundamental distinction between drug use and medication use.** Medicine, in this context, is that which is prescribed and monitored only by a qualified doctor or nurse practitioner experienced in the treatment of alcohol and substance use disorders.

2. **Medication is considered under the umbrella of self-care versus self-harm.** For opioid addictions, suboxone, subutex, and methadone are used to limit the harm of unabated opioid addiction, which is life-threatening. It is considered a useful measure of significant harm reduction.

3. There are often underlying conditions like depression, anxiety, PTSD, or bipolar, for which psychiatric medicine can help take some of the edge off their symptoms and are safe and not habit-forming. Since one of the drivers of substance use is the **self-medicating of these conditions, shifting to the proper professional oversight and prescribing of them is an important step toward better self-care.** Ironically, when offered these medicines, many users immediately become excessively concerned that they are going to get hooked on these medicines, become dependent on them, and get terrible unwanted side effects.

4. Many will insist on being provided a side effect list so they can weigh the risks and benefits. When I ask them if they have ever looked up the side effects of alcohol, fentanyl, cocaine, benzos or even pot, they often smile and begin to appreciate the irony.

5. **Benzodiazepines** like Xanax, Ativan, and Klonopin are commonly used in the treatment of anxiety disorders, but in my view, can only play a limited role in the treatment of alcohol and substance use disorders—which is specifically the treatment of acute withdrawal from alcohol, substances or from benzos themselves. Benzodiazepines are also very helpful in the treatment of acute anxiety, where no possibility of habit formation will occur, as in the treatment of the anxiety about flying on an airplane. To take one pill on the flight out and another on the return trip can help relieve the anxiety without risk of habit formation and is not a problem. However, these medications are generally a disaster in the treatment of chronic and everyday anxiety and should be avoided for that purpose, as they are habit-forming and invariably compound the treatment of the substance use. **Bottom line: if you need a medication for everyday anxiety, don't make it a benzo or any other habit-forming medication. Mindfulness calls on us to be selective and only put into our bodies that which is beneficial and keep out that which can be harmful.**

6. **ADHD meds**: While there is high co-morbidity between alcohol and substance use disorders and ADD or ADHD conditions, ADHD meds are truly most beneficial in childhood when they are most needed and before the onset of the substance use. The chief ADHD symptoms for which substance users want ADHD meds are distractibility and inability to focus. These symptoms also occur in the depression, anxiety, PTSD, and bipolar conditions which are almost always invariably co-occur with substance use. Some of these symptoms are also the result of brain changes that occur in the brain as a result of the repeated substance use and lessen considerably once the substance use has stopped. Finally, since substance use is unfortunately a relapsing disorder, prescribing these meds provides yet another substance than can be abused. Moreover, having these medications in their systems when they relapse only confounds the treatment of their withdrawal and recovery. Lastly, mindfulness training helps us to appreciate that **everyone's amygdala is in an ADHD state.**

The amygdala is the area of the brain where distractibility, impulsivity and difficulty sitting still and paying attention are generated.

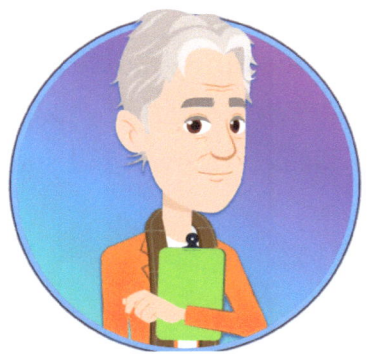

Recent studies have shown that shortly after Cocaine use, the amygdala area is activated, while at the same time there is a measurable decreased blood flow to the prefrontal cortex that can last for weeks. This means that there is some part of our attentional problems that is self-created by the substance use itself, and for which users are now seeking ADHD meds to alleviate. It's like drinking coffee before bedtime and then complaining of not being able to sleep. Our prefrontal cortex is our override system for our distractibility, and by adulthood, sufficient myelination has occurred in the prefrontal cortex to allow it to strengthen and strategize a plan to reign in the distractibility and learn ways to compensate for the amygdala's lack of focus without relying on a medication that will likely complicate their treatment.

7. **Anti-Craving Medications:** Because alcohol and substance use disorders are life-threatening conditions, I urge that the use of anti-craving meds such as Naltrexone, Vivitrol, and Antabuse be a part of the treatment discussion. My approach is that anything that has a chance of helping without causing harm should be considered.

8. **Medicate or Educate:** Often the mindset of a user is that their brain is missing a chemical necessary for their happiness, and they cop an attitude toward the Doc: "Well if you prescribe what I really need then I won't get it on the street", which, of course, also means that "If you don't prescribe me what I want, I will just get it on the streets!" I see **our job is to not just medicate, but to educate** and tactfully help them recognize that **their mindset is part of the problem**. Most of the brain requires absolutely no different add-on chemicals. In fact, the best part of our brain, our prefrontal cortex, like a stallion, needs to be

exercised more to release its natural chemicals.

The educational framing also invites our patients to see themselves to be more than just patients but also students – that is, not just in treatment to have something done to them, to be treated, detoxed, prescribed medications, but pro-actively defining what it is they need to learn – developing coping skills about addiction, about the brain, and about themselves to recover and stay recovered.

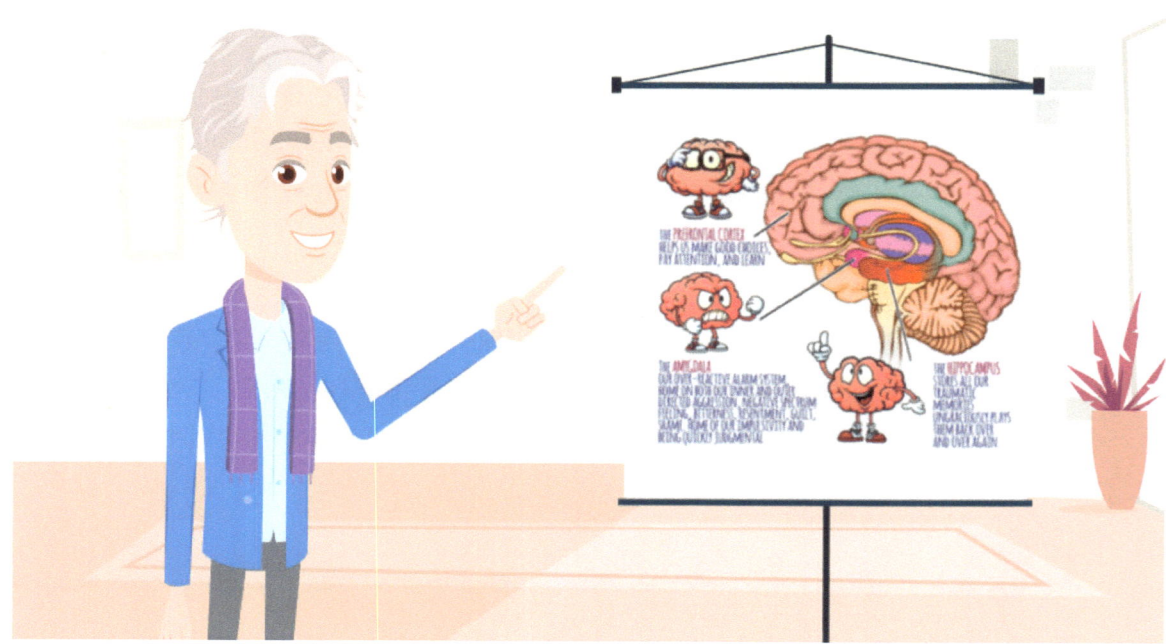

Understanding the Prefrontal Cortex

In 1848, Phineas Gage was a twenty-five-year-old well-respected and well-liked railroad construction foreman, who was involved in an accident laying rail that ironically would help us begin to understand the neuronal tracks that evolution had laid down in our prefrontal cortex. Phineas was managing a crew laying new track in Vermont for the railroad expansion and using a tamping iron—a 3.5 foot long, 1.25 inch wide metal rod weighing 13 pounds—to tamp down dynamite powder with sand in the side of a mountain to create a path for new railroad track. When the tamping iron hit a rock, it flicked a spark that ignited an explosion sending the tamping iron through his cheek and through his prefrontal cortex, landing 100 yards away with some of his prefrontal cortex attached to it.

While Gage miraculously survived this ordeal, within 3 months his behavior changed radically and his sense of responsibility toward himself and others deteriorated markedly, and he was impaired in his ability to make decisions and choices conducive to his betterment. In a more recent 1992 version of this story, famed music composer David Foster inadvertently struck Broadway star, Ben Vareen, who, while

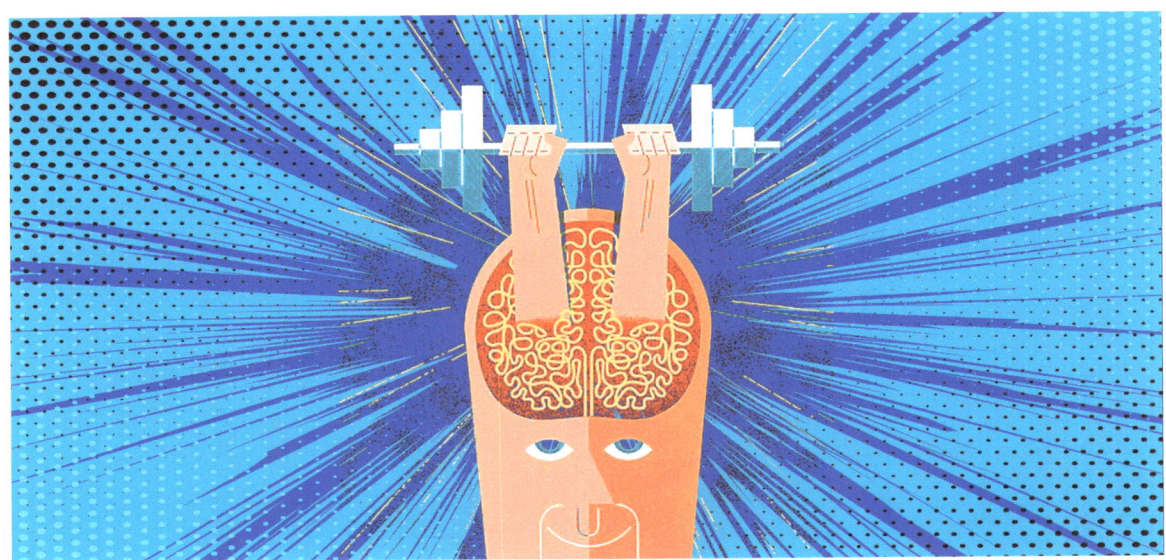

walking along the Malibu highway, suffered a stroke that impaired his ability to act in a self-protective manner, and he suddenly veered into the highway. The story has a paradoxical happy ending though, because it seems the stroke was caused by the aneurysm bleed—which was only discovered when he arrived at the hospital for the treatment of his car accident injuries and the required brain scans, which in the end likely saved his life.

It is reasonable to conclude that the prefrontal cortex plays a crucial role in our ability to make decisions and act in ways that are advantageous to our survival and future. However, all human beings, way too often, do not act in their best interest—thankfully not because of suffering a tamping iron blow to the prefrontal cortex. It seems that some other factors or psychological issues must drive us to underutilize or block the oversight and guidance that this crucial brain area is capable of providing.

Our prefrontal cortex is by far the best and most advanced part our brain. It is not only fabulous, as it is, but it is also open for development. It is educable and expandable. We all under-utilize this crucial part of our cortical real estate. It is the home of our best selves, the part that can learn to turn lemons into lemonade. It is the great synthesizer and integrator of our lives gathering up all our failings and disappointments, helping us to compost our heartaches into the soil of our future growth, inspiring us to move on from, and away from, our negative-self preoccupations. If the measure of our maturity is our evolving capacity to suppress impulsive and inappropriate behavior, it is to our prefrontal cortex that we turn to enhance and develop this capacity.

I was sitting on my deck one recent summer night and watched a tiny bug move across the deck railing. I wondered what kinds of awareness it possessed. Could it see, respond to hot and cold, could it hear, taste, smell? I thought about how tiny its brain was and how it had to make its way in the world with such a small engine.

I surmised that it must be efficiently using every square inch of its brain's real estate. Then I thought about our human brain and all the additional kinds of awareness we possess. I also thought how much of our brain's real estate is underutilized and the untapped potential this allows us.

Understanding the Prefrontal Cortex

There are 7 key metaphors that can illuminate and help us understand better the capabilities our prefrontal cortex affords us: grasping hand, tool chest, CEO, orchestra conductor, the loving and protective parent, the gardener, and the musical instrument.

Our Prefrontal Cortex Allows Us to Grasp Abstract Concepts.

Piaget was a Swiss developmental psychologist who helped us to learn about our ability to grasp and utilize higher level abstract concepts. While an animal's brain can clearly generate the movements of walking, it cannot generate the idea of walking, never mind the idea of shoes to help protect the feet from harm or provide comfort and stability. Only a human being can appreciate that **there is nothing as powerful as a good idea.**

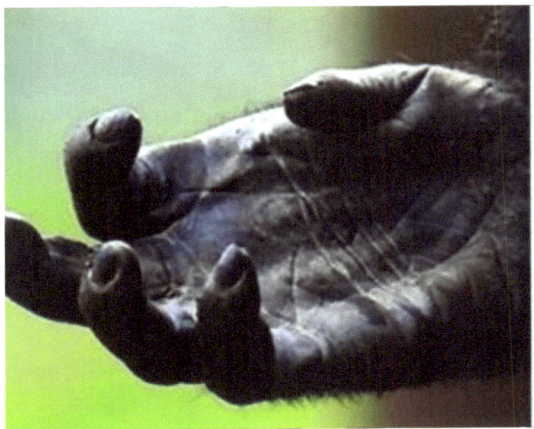 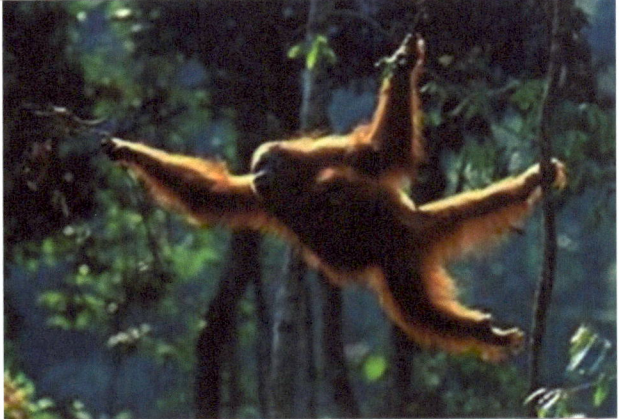

From an evolutionary perspective, we can see that the curved prehensile hand shape of monkeys was well adapted for grasping branches, allowing ready access to food and escape from danger.

We can also understand that the functioning of **our prefrontal cortex was shaped so to speak, not to grasp branches but to grasp ideas**—such as the concepts of illness, well-being, inner peace, awe, and love that can't be held in our hands but which can mentally transport us to that which truly sustains us at another level.

Brian L. Ackerman, M.D.

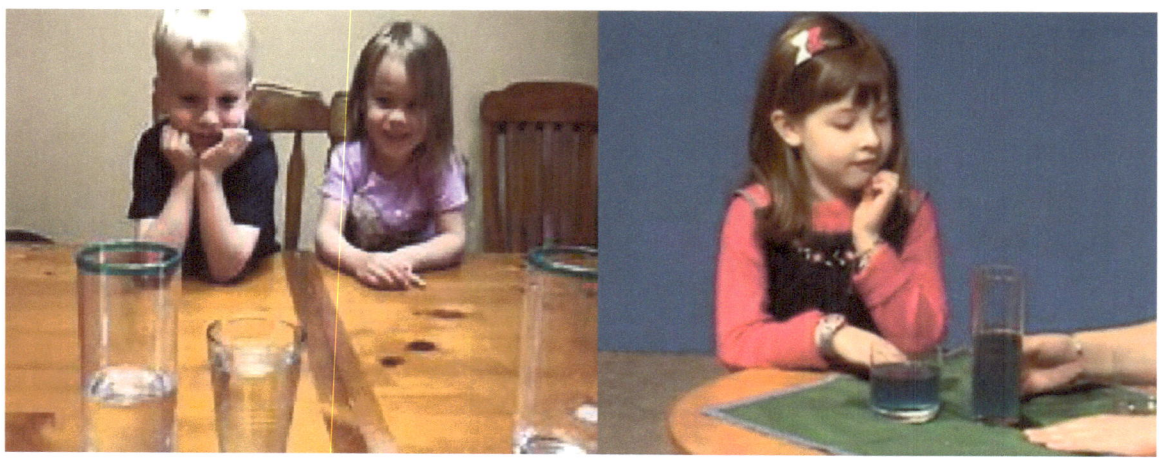

Piaget helped us understand that it took a certain degree of brain development before a child's brain could grasp the distinction between size and quantity—which differ by their level of abstraction: quantity represents a higher level of abstraction requiring a higher cognitive function, over size.

I remember presenting Piaget's studies on children's evolving capacity to grasp abstract ideas to a group at a wellness fair when the person assigned to run my PowerPoint presentation came up to me afterwards and told me that that my presentation helped him understand something about his intellectually handicapped kid brother he had never understood before. He said that in money games, his brother would always pick 4 single dollar bills over a 5-dollar bill because, as he understood better now—to his brother, 4 bills was more than 1 bill, and the symbol and significance of the numeral 5 was beyond his grasp.

It seems our capacity to grasp higher-level concepts continues and develops throughout our lives, and this is precisely where we need to put our energies. Rather than devoting our efforts to getting our amygdala to shut up, we can better devote our energies to getting our prefrontal cortex more fully up-and-running, and do more of what it does best: see the big picture, see ourselves accurately, and with love and compassion, care for ourselves and our future, protecting us from harm. Most of all, like an alert security guard, it can help us **learn not to become hijacked by the amygdala.**

Understanding the Prefrontal Cortex

One of the crucial questions we address with folks in treatment and recovery is **why alcohol and substance users fail to grasp the many dangerous consequences of their use**, and why if they are capable of grasping it, do they still seem to not get that they are **using poisons** that can and will, harm them, poison their body and brain, interfere with their capacity to work, poison their relationships, harm others, leave them hating themselves, and render them unable to care for themselves, nevermind anyone else.

Alcohol and substance treatment staff are called upon to help these devoted self-injurers recognize the severity of these self-injurious impulses and behaviors, without for one moment buying into the nonsense that these folks are operating under their own volition. One could imagine the amygdala being a cult and its possessor under its spell. Mindfulness training invites all to learn about the brain and learn how to access and use the best parts of it. It also calls on us to become more aware of the amygdala's straight jacket confinement and learn to **liberate ourselves from its spell.**

The **PREFRONTAL CORTEX is a TOOL that contains to key that unlocks the handcuffs that keep us tied to our amygdala and our substance use.**

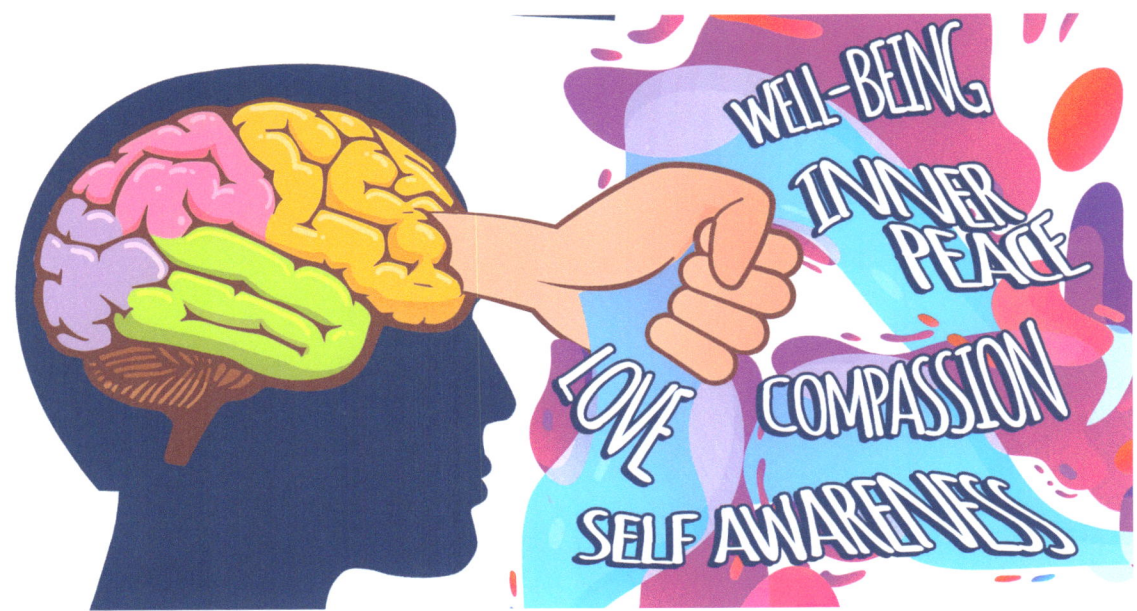

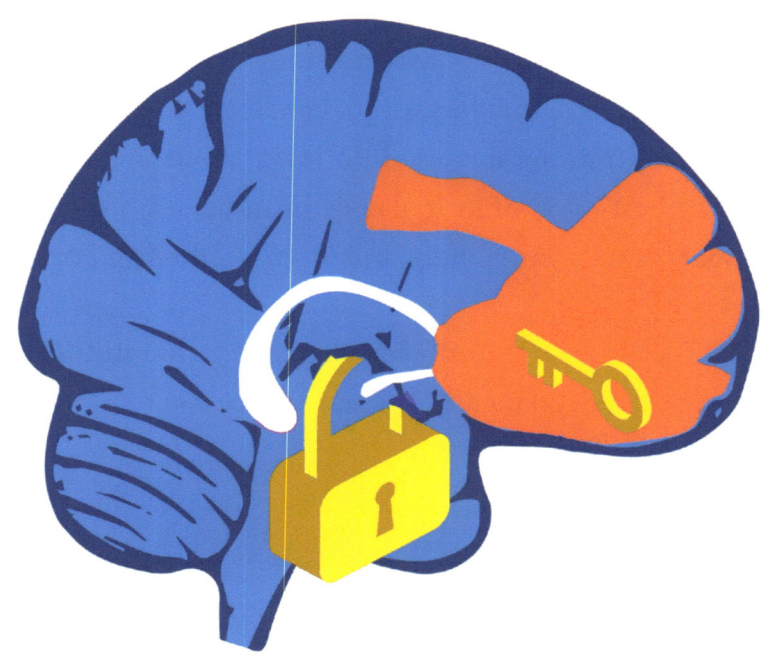

The **PRE-FRONTAL CORTEX** is a tool

It contains the key to unlock what keeps us tied to our Amygdala and our substance use.

Understanding the Prefrontal Cortex

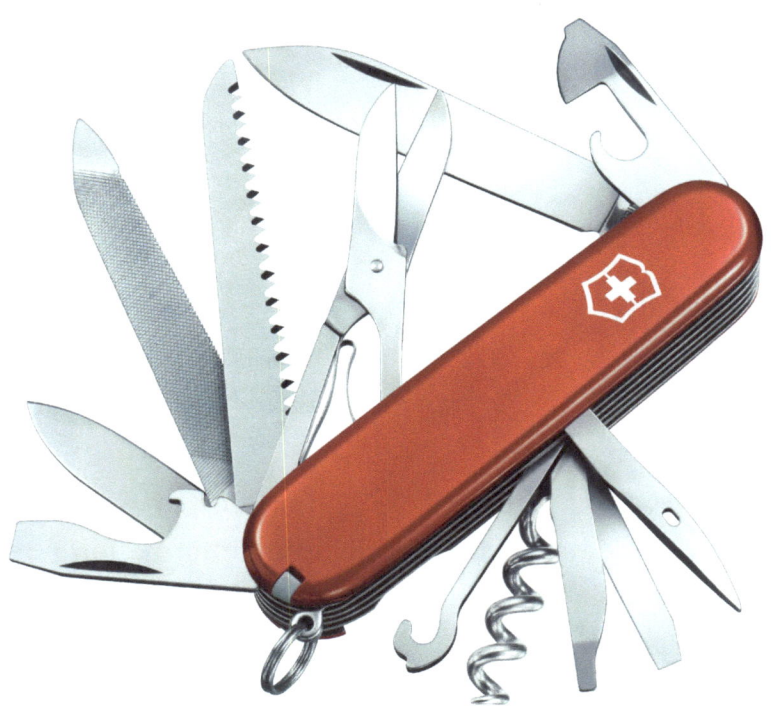

Blade of Awareness and Witnessing

Blade of Perspective, Inner Vision & Self-Reflection Blade of Grasping, Realizing Significance

Blade of Self-care and Self & Other-Protection Blade of Self Worth

Blade of *Humor*

Blade of our Higher Intelligence

Blade of Higher Reasoning, Strategizing & Problem-Solving Blade of Calmness, Inner peace and Joy.

Blade of Hopefulness & Future Focus. Blade of Gratitude, Glad to be alive Blade of AWE.

Blade of Resiliency and Determination Blade of Love & Compassion.

Blade of Insight into Self & Others

Blades of Reasoning Intelligently about Cause & Effect Blade of Making Distinctions without Judgment

Blade of Determining Priorities Blade of Future planning Blade of Wisdom

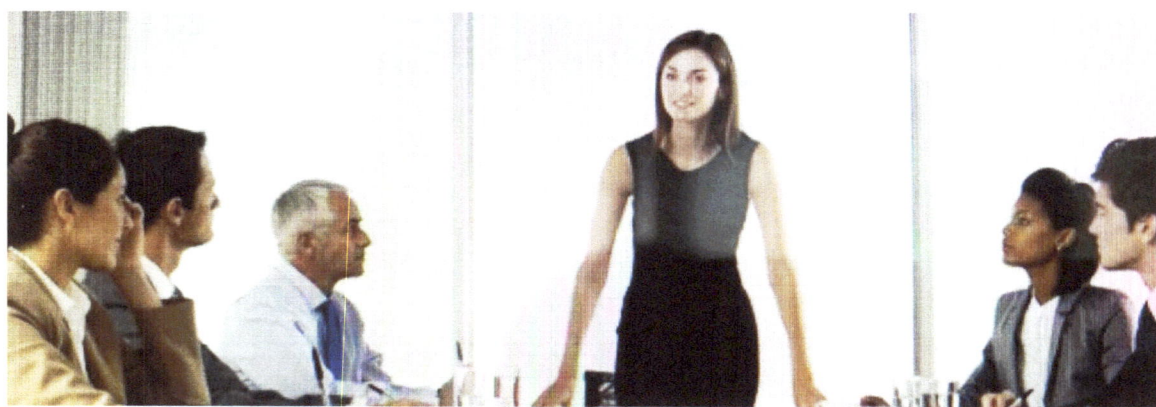

The prefrontal cortex is like the **CEO of the company** with all the other brain modules acting as middle managers and gathering information for the CEO to be discussed and reasoned amongst the team, but is prepared for the final executive decision to be made by the CEO—who makes the final decision even when the amygdala is heckling or creating a roadblock.

The prefrontal cortex is also like the **conductor of an orchestra** with other brain modules as the instruments which highlight the purpose of conductor to know the beauty of the music and direct the instruments to play together in such a way as to create harmony. The conductor also knows the potentially beneficial role of the amygdala as the instrument of the drum which can keep the beat and add points of emphasis, but which can also—if becomes too loud—can actually disturb and at times, drown out the music.

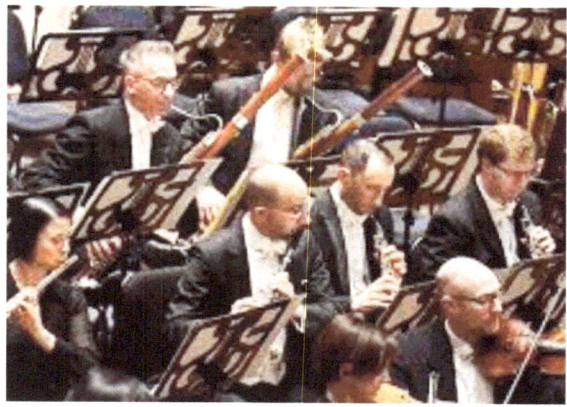
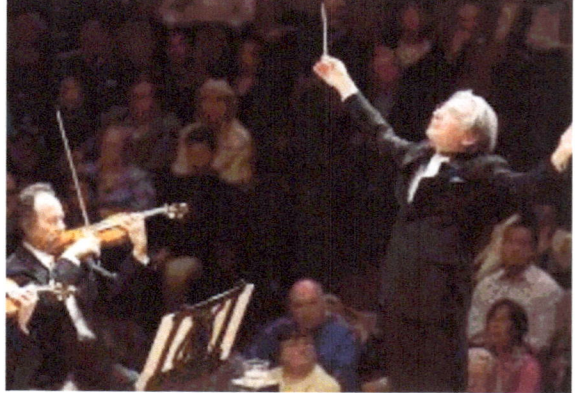

Understanding the Prefrontal Cortex

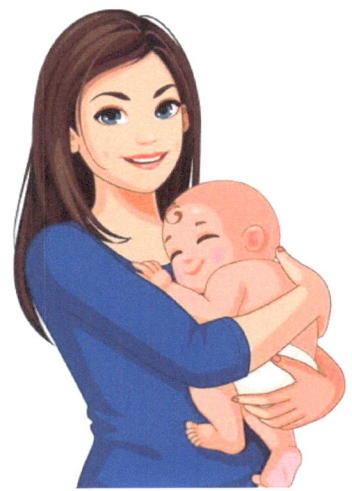

The prefrontal cortex is also like a **loving parent** attending to their children's essential needs for body and spiritual nutrition, while protecting them from mental and physical harm.

The prefrontal cortex can act like our **mental gardener** who knows that there are fabulous vegetables and fruits to be grown and picked, but also weeds that need to be pulled so that the desired growth can occur.

Finally, the prefrontal cortex can be imagined as a **musician** playing the brain (an amazing instrument). Whether or not I learn to play guitar or piano is a matter of taste, choice, and interest. But it seems that learning to "play the brain", so to speak, may actually be necessary for us to find inner peace and contentment.

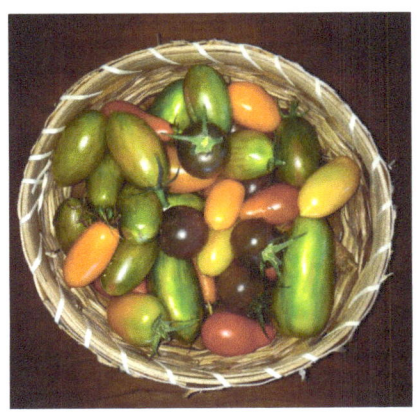
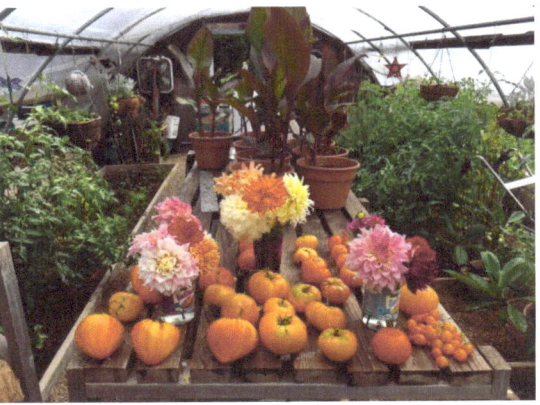

Brian L. Ackerman, M.D.

If we consider the fine finger or vocal adjustments needed to get the most harmonious sounds out of an instrument, or think about all the practice needed to produce a quality sound out of a musical instrument, we can begin to imagine the inner harmony we might be able to create as a mindfulness practice approach of learning how to "play the brain". Fundamental to this approach is to envision our brain as an amazing instrument capable of producing a kind of "music" that can truly inspire.

Mindfulness emphasizes the upstairs and downstairs aspects of the brain in order to understand better our psychological struggles, more so than the left-right hemisphere differences of the brain. To help ourselves, we can learn to better utilize more of our upstairs cortex. This makes sense, as the upstairs is the most evolved area of our brain. It is not a coincidence that a fundamental adage of AA is one "step" at a time, and that both dimensions of taking a step: understanding it as a concept and metaphor, what it means to takes steps toward ones goals, as well as the physical enactment of step-taking all coming from the upstairs cortex. While this may not be our "Staircase to Heaven," it does appear to be our staircase of our inner peace and well-being.

Left-right distinctions are especially useful when our brain has suffered blunt trauma or a stroke. In my teachings I do sing the praises of our prefrontal upstairs cortex, and provide warning signs for our downstairs amygdala, but I am not trying to say that the upstairs of the brain is good and that the downstairs is bad.

The lowest part of our brain—our brainstem—which functions like the utility room of a large commercial building, is simply amazing. It keeps our heart ticking, our lungs breathing, and our body temperature and glucose levels carefully regulated.

Similarly, our cerebellum—which keeps us physically balanced—is another fabulous lower and more primitive area of our brain. I prefer the distinction of useful or beneficial versus harmful or counterproductive as a framework for a comparative assessment of our brain areas. Some areas are simply more beneficial than others; some are more beneficial in certain contexts and less so than others. In the darkness, for example, our ability to smell a fire with our olfactory cortex may be life-saving, while during the day, seeing it with our visual cortex or hearing it with our auditory cortex may be what saves us.

Understanding the Prefrontal Cortex

Much is also said of whether or not we only use ten to twenty percent of our brain. My perspective on this is that if our brain stem can perform all its functions by utilizing only ten percent of its capacity, that's terrific because that allows energy resources to be shifted elsewhere. From an efficiency perspective, mindfulness teaches us that our amygdala area is an energy waster as we can easily become consumed by our negative thoughts and feelings. It makes sense that we would want to divert more of our energy resources to our prefrontal cortex.

Our prefrontal cortex can find a way to circumvent our anger and negative spectrum thoughts and feelings so we are not flooded by them, which might be a wise choice by diverting or circumventing negativity. If our prefrontal cortex can function like a dam, and then actually convert the adverse flooding energy of anger and anxiety into electrical power, then we may well have discovered the secret to enlightenment: converting negative destructive energy into a positive, useful benefit. Mindfulness teaches us to be aware of where our psychic energy is flowing and to make adjustments accordingly.

It seems we are utilizing perhaps as much of eighty percent of our amygdala and only twenty percent of our prefrontal cortex. Our well-being may be tied to the degree that we can learn to reverse this ratio.

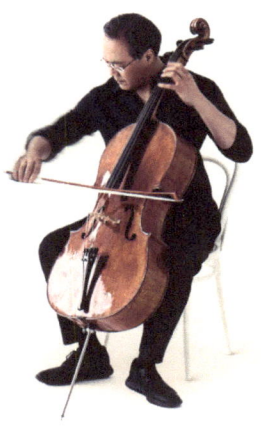

MENTAL WASTE

In the mindfulness groups I run, I bring in a **waste basket** with the sign on it called: **Mental Waste**, so that the **prop** can remind us how accustomed we are to throwing out physical stuff that no longer serves a purpose. In mindfulness training, we realize we need to also figure out a way to **throw out our mental trash also while also realizing how much of it accumulates.**

The following are the instructions to go with this exercise:

Please deposit here all your negative thoughts and feelings you have about yourself: your feelings of defectiveness, deficiencies, and disconnectedness. Please deposit here any feeling that you do not belong or that you are not worthy. Please deposit here your anger, resentment, bitterness, criticism of yourself and others. Please deposit here all of your self-harming impulses, and urges, desires, and cravings to use alcohol or substances or to act in any way contrary to your well-being, health, and best interests. Please deposit here all of your tendencies to compare yourself to others.

Once you have freed yourself of, and deposited all of this mental waste, you will begin to see the buds of your inner peace and your self-worth. There is an effort you must make to feel better, to remove the mental waste that so burdens you and to nurture and care for the buds of your healthy spirit, and your uniqueness—which is buried under the waste and held back because of it.

The consequence of not making the effort is that you will continue spending way too much time feeling lousy.

Let's consider for a moment what are the built-in mechanisms we have that can serve to release any of this mental waste and how effective they are in accomplishing this task.

Here's what I have identified: Laughter, dreams, tears, exercise, sports, yoga, music (both listening and playing), reading, writing, learning, having meaningful conversations with friends, family, and therapists, going to the theater, plays, movies, playing and having fun, being out in nature.

The good news is that each of these activities helps a little and doing all of them helps a lot. The bad news is that even if we faithfully do them all, we are still left with suitcases full of mental waste that still needs to be dumped and released for us to feel well.

Mindfulness Training was specifically developed to help be aware of this and to help us roll up our sleeves and deliberately remove as much of the residual mental waste as we can.

So yes, to access inner peace, laugh your brains out often, dream away, stretch, exercise, get out into nature, have meaningful conversations, read, study, learn, listen to and if possible learn to play music, and find ways to have fun that doesn't put yourself in harm's way.

But then also do the mental homework, the mental flossing. Be humbled by the negative mental flooding of thoughts and feelings that recur out of the slightest provocation and develop the tools of awareness and selectivity to not become hijacked by it.

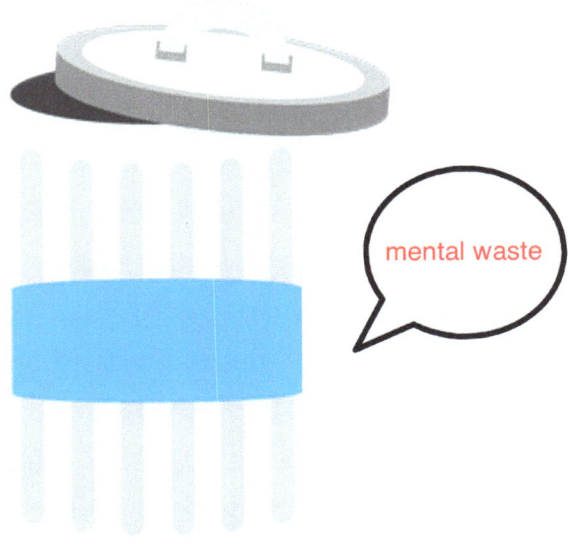

ARE YOU READY TO MAKE THE EFFORT?

Cravings

All cravings are not equally beneficial. Different brain regions might have desires and appetites for very different things. One brain area we often jokingly refer to as our "sweet tooth". Most alcohol and substance users report they have rather intense alcohol or substance cravings. But this use of the term 'cravings' does not make sense to me. As a physician, I understand a **true craving to be for that which our body truly needs to help it come into physiological balance.** So, if we are dehydrated, we understand thirst (a water craving) or a salt craving to replace and rebalance the water and salt lost through sweat. But our bodies and brains do not intrinsically need or want alcohol and even when this desire is self-created by repeated use. Only a small part of the brain has any interest in it, while **most of the brain wants nothing to do with these so called "cravings".**

If the parents of six children ask the kids what they want for dinner, and the baby cries out for "formula", that clearly is not going to satisfy the other five kids. So too, when one tiny brain region cries out for drugs or alcohol, we need to think about what our other brain regions want and need. We also need to get creative about what we "feed" our amygdala to get it to quiet down. Remember, we are not trying to feed it steak to fatten it up. If it were our dog who was restless even after chowing down, we might give it a rubber bone to chew on to keep it occupied and calm.

The awareness and distinction that different brain regions may well "crave" very different things was further brought home to me when I did a psychiatric evaluation with a woman who had attended one of my mindfulness groups in an IOP program. Two days later when I ran into her in the hallway, she remarked: "You're the mindfulness doc!". I asked her, "How did you like the group?" She said, 'I loved it!" and went on say: 'I love to learn!' and then added: **"I crave knowledge!"**

Now, I had never heard anyone before make reference to a knowledge craving but it made sense to me because it is referring to something we truly need: knowledge and learning, and *we can imagine that these intense higher quality desires as the 'cravings' of our prefrontal cortex; while a candy or drug craving is vintage amygdala.*

I invite alcohol and substance users when they are being overwhelmed by their drug cravings, to ask themselves what is it that they truly crave, and what is truly out of balance?

The next mindfulness training craving strategy is to learn to disconnect the sense of "I" from the lower craving. If it is an amygdala craving, we learn to say: "It is my amygdala that craves drugs, leaving my authentic "I" free to truly prefer fresh air, spring water, or a walk in nature.

In mindfulness training, we learn to reserve the use of "I" for the prefrontal cortex and only for that which we truly want, need, and can benefit from. In that sense, the statement "I crave knowledge", can be a very accurate statement, while the statement; "I crave alcohol", is not.

Martin Buber, a noted religious philosopher, wrote about the I-Thou relationship—a paradigm that can help us better understand and imagine, our relationship with God. Mindfulness training helps us to better understand our relationship with ourselves, and it introduces the **concept of the I-It relationship** to help us better understand and imagine with our amygdala and our relationship to it.

This I-It distinction is an essential teaching of Mindfulness Training and helps us learn not to over-identify with aspects of ourselves that are just small parts. For example, I think of myself as *having* a gallbladder, but I never think of myself *as* a gallbladder. I can learn that bile is in the gallbladder, but I never think of myself as bile. Or, I can think of myself as having a pancreas, but never think of myself as a pancreas. So too, I can learn that I have an amygdala but learn to disidentify with this small part of the brain. I have anger, fear, anxiety, distractibility irritability, impulsivity, negative thoughts in my amygdala, in me; but they are not me. I have an amygdala in me; but I am not my amygdala, and I am not what comes from my amygdala. This separation of the I from the it, helps us protect and preserve our well-being and sense of true self, when our amygdala acts up.

Alcoholics Anonymous has, by far, the best track record in treating the alcohol and substance-using population than any other treatment modality, and I encourage all my patients to participate. For so many, this grass roots, self-help organization

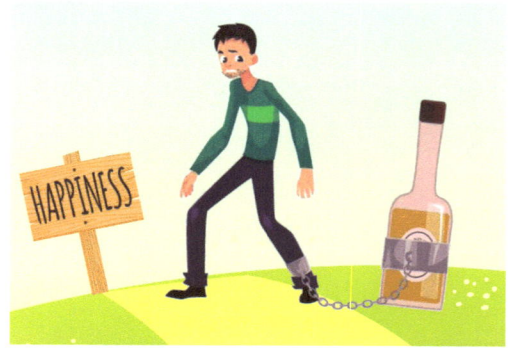

has been a game changer and provides crucial lifelines to millions in the darkest of their despair. While their program has twelve steps, many participants don't buy into the entire AA way of thinking, but they participate anyway. Some don't believe, for example—in a higher power. One of the many ingredients to AA's success that has been identified, is that they offer people who feel like misfits—like they don't belong—an opportunity for membership: a place where they can go and belong.

"Hello, my name is Joe, I'm an alcoholic." The group recognizes this as a crucial stage of recovery: admitting to having a problem that they have lost control of. But in the background, we are reminded of the Woody Allen joke: "I wouldn't want to be a part of a group that would have me as a member!"

Mindfulness training takes issue with identifying oneself by one's substance use. "I'm an alcoholic" may be the ticket of admission to AA. However, while AA is free, this ticket of 'admission', from a mindfulness perspective is way too costly. When someone has cancer, for example, they never identify themselves by the cancer. They say "I have cancer", not "I am cancer". Mindfulness invites us to realize the club that we are already members of is that of being human. Within a part of their mind lies their psychological cancer, but they are much more than their substance use. Mindfulness teaches that it is the non-substance using part of their brain—the non-substance desiring part of their upper mind—that will drive their recovery, and allowing themselves to be open to a higher power, or the power of others' support, of the underutilized power of their own brain and any combination of the above is crucial.

The I-It relationship offers an alternative: "I have a part of my brain and mind that is alcoholic," leaving the part of my brain and mind that is not alcoholic free to grab the steering wheel of my life, which includes hauling my butt over to an AA Meeting (in person or remotely) to find some more effective way to keep that part of my brain and mind that is alcoholic in check.

MENTAL DIALYSIS

This is the core mindfulness homework activity that I have all my mindfulness group participants do as their weekly homework assignment. To get the most out of what you are learning about in this book, **I highly recommend you start doing this homework on a daily basis**. It can also be used like a journal. Whenever you spot a lower level thought, feeling, or impulse, write it down on paper under the heading of toxic lower level. Conversely, when you become aware of a higher-level thought, feeling, or impulse jot that down in its proper column.

The purpose of this exercise is to help free the upper mind of the mental muck that comes from the lower mind. Keep a **daily diary** of whatever thoughts, feelings, impulses, pre-occupations, or worries that you have become aware of, and mark them down in the appropriate columns. This sorting into columns is mental filtration. With this activity, we are mentally separating our thoughts, feelings and impulses: those that benefit us from those that don't. This is the function of what a filter does: the desired coffee is allowed through, the grinds are held back; oxygen is retained, CO_2 is let out; useful thoughts extracted, counterproductive ones are held back.

MENTAL DIALYSIS

A Mindfulness Exercise Developed by Brian L. Ackerman MD

Purpose: To free our higher and best nature of the mental muck that comes from the lower mind: The Amygdala

What to do: Keep a daily diary of whatever thoughts, feelings, impulses, pre-occupations, worries, and self-defeating behaviors that you can become aware of and write down in the appropriate column.

By doing this we are learning how filter out of our psyche that which entangles us in feeling lousy and in making unwise decisions.

LOWER LEVEL	UPPER LEVEL

EXAMPLES

LOWER LEVEL	UPPER LEVEL
The thought: There is no use. **The feeling:** I feel depressed, bored. **The impulse:** I just want to use so badly!	I am sick of having my life run by drugs. I want my kids back. I want to have a life and I am going to get mine back. I realize my drug use is a dead end street and I do not want to die. I actually do care!

What follows are copies of a few of my actual patient-completed weekly homework assignments which are handed in at the beginning of the group, then read aloud, and discussed. Please note that the columns are variously referred to lower versus higher level, amygdala vs prefrontal cortex, negative vs positive, and it vs I. It is the making of these kinds of distinctions that is key to the success of mental dialysis.

Lower Level thinking	Upper Level thinking
It has been bored a lot recently. And not too excited about 2020	I decided to organize a vision board with a completion date of 2/3/2020
The mentorship experience has been heavy and expensive. It feels a little taken advantage of by the young girl I am mentoring.	I know I need to be patient and let things develop. It may improve in time with effort and energy

Negative	Positive
It is holding me back in sadness, self hatred, unclear thoughts, self doubt, shame and guilt. I have battled with these thoughts for so long. It has become my belief system.	Don't let these thoughts & feelings define who I am. I want to gain forward momentum in life. Be kinder to self. Be Patient to self.
After Christmas it had the crash of sadness and guilt for feeling bad. I have had a lot of losses to live through. It did not let me grieve.	I want to feel everyday is a gift. I know life is fragile. I want to take better care of myself and find myself again.
It It being my lack of motivation, energy, self-worth, and the fear gets in the way of doing things that are best for me. It keeps me stuck.	**I** I need to look at the steps I am taking to change and recover. I am getting help to do this. I want to feel hopeful and have some joy in my life.

Mental Dialysis

It

My brother was talking to me about lowering the heat during the day. He brought up that he was not home during the day. Then my "Stinkin Thinking" responded by accusing him of trying to make me feel guilty about having the heat to high during the day. He responded by saying he hated my victim shit and trying to talk to me. I walked away hurt and angry.

I

I sat with my emotions and after I calmed down, I realized it was not my brother's intentions to make me feel guilty, that was my "Stinkin Thinking".

Lower Psyche	Higher Psyche
It gave me a bad day. It made me so depressed that I haven't seen my granddaughter in months. It made me feel like my son hated me.	I decided to make the first move. I called my son and told him how I felt. He asked me if I would like to spend some time with my granddaughter. I was absolutely thrilled. He brought them over and also gave me a big hug. My granddaughter ran up to me and said that they loved me. It made me feel so loved that I couldn't put it into words how wonderful I felt.
It gave me a terrible night. It wouldn't let me sleep.	I did some breathing exercises and also some meditation. I soon calmed down and was finally able to sleep.

Mental Dialysis

Lower Psyche	Higher Psyche
It made me full of anxiety when I went to to the play around with my daughters and grandsons. It made me want to go home.	Instead of going home I thought to myself not to let it spoil my time with my grandsons. I was then calmed down and had a great day with them
It made me a nervous wreck when I went to the nursing home to see my mom ~~all the times kids~~. She was sound asleep. My sisters and I tried so hard to wake her up nothing worked. It made me worry about her	I calmed myself down and said to myself that she was 94 years old and she would be alright the next time I go to see her.

MENTAL DIALYSIS

A Mindfulness Exercise Developed by Brian L. Ackerman MD

Purpose: To free the upper mind of the mental muck that comes from the lower mind.

What to do: Keep a daily diary of whatever thoughts, feelings, impulses, pre-occupations, worries that you can become aware of and write down in the appropriate column.

LOWER LEVEL	UPPER LEVEL
○ I'm not kind	○ I know that when I'm at my best I care about people and mankind.
○ I deserve whatever I get if I caught some STD	
○ people pretend to like me but secretly hate my guts	○ I could change the world for the better w/ tenacity and focus
○ I'm tired of fucking up my life	○ Even though it hurts its best to let people go when I know they are not good for me.
○ I'm not as smart as	

MENTAL DIALYSIS

I think or other people think

When I was assaulted I deserved it.

They will never catch my assailant.

My father is keeping me away from my dying mother

I can achieve anything I put my mind to.

Duel Diagnosis

We are in the home stretch now on our brain journey and in our quest to understand ourselves and make changes for the better.

Our goal is quite specific and clear: to learn to make wiser choices that are based on self-care and self-protection while keeping our eyes on the prize: the diligent pursuit of our health and well-being.

Despite the numerous times we have made the same mistake repeatedly, **we are all capable of learning new things** especially if we feel inspired by a good teacher to do so—and I hope I have been that for you. I hope you will take the time to read and re-read this book often, as you won't absorb all of it the first time. I also hope you will do the journal homework outlined in the book, as this is the essential homework of mental dialysis. By now you understand how essential it is for all of us to free our minds of mental toxicity—to free our identities from it. And because this mental toxicity rebuilds daily, we must take the time every day, to mental floss to free our minds of negative thoughts, feelings, and impulses that will continue to pop up.

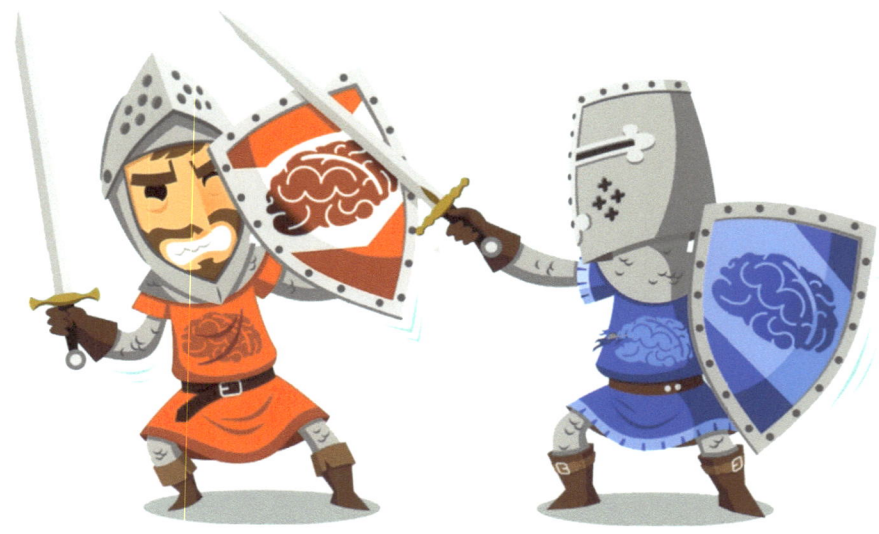

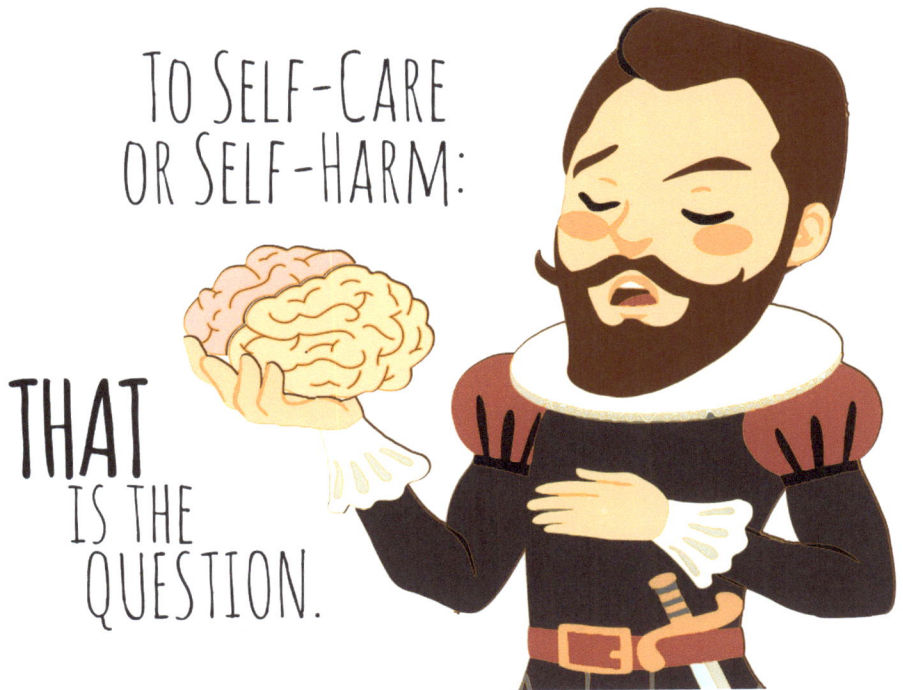

A diagnosis is a label, and labels are only helpful if they are accurate and beneficial. Most diagnostic labels are inaccurate, while some are actually harmful.

The label most alcohol and substance users give themselves is:

"I'm an addict." However, the "diagnostic label" I suggest we all use for ourselves, first and foremost, is that we are HUMAN! Then I encourage all of us to **better understand our condition: being human.** This then leads us to the next "diagnosis" that I introduce in mindfulness training called **duel diagnosis, which I consider to be at the core of our "human condition".**

I like the term: **duel diagnosis** over the more usual term dual diagnosis for several reasons. Firstly, I view alcohol and substance use disorders on a continuum of mental health disorders. In this book, I have articulated the view that alcohol and substance use is indeed a mental health problem because it is a form of self-injury. **When we have our mental health, we do not go out of our way to harm ourselves and we really do care about the consequences of our actions on ourselves as well as others.** We have also learned about the adverse effect of having negative thoughts,

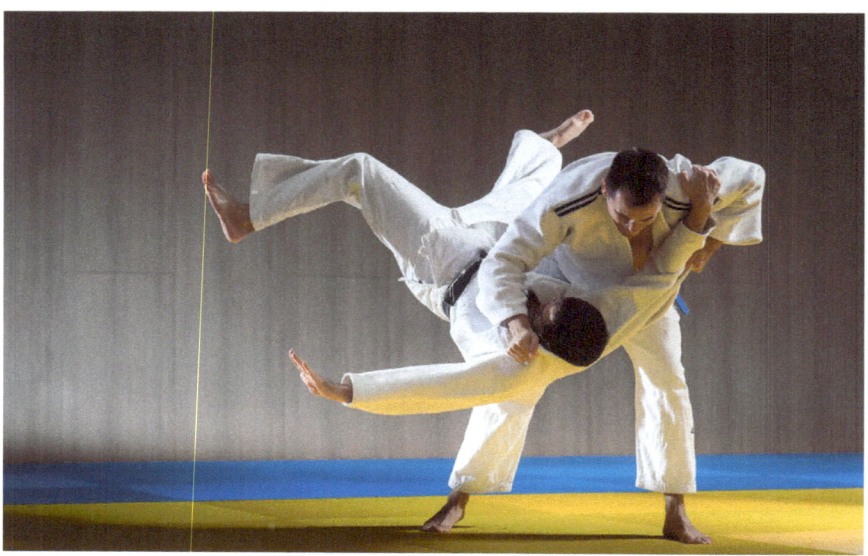

feelings, and impulses swirling around in our minds. While we don't go out of our way to find these negative thoughts, like bees—they surely find us, and do they ever sting. They love to nest in anxious, depressed, and angry moods, and we have to learn to be less hospitable to them.

I used to think that the "whistle" to begin a duel was "On guard", like "On your mark." Later I learned it was "Engage". We want people to truly "engage" with life, and the thesis of this work is that to engage with life optimally, one has to first successfully engage with one's amygdala.

Often in the mindfulness groups I run, I use props like fake swords and role playing to help bring to awareness the intensity of this inner duel. I have one group member play the role of their prefrontal cortex, while another group member plays the role of the amygdala. You would be surprised how quickly people learn to tell their amygdala with rather convincing authority to " Stick a sock in it!" The lines of their Amygdala are like, "Who do you think you're kidding, you're never going to stick with sobriety!", while they are play-acted, the lines come so quickly as if memorized from real life.

This exercise is also to help underscore a central theme of mindfulness training: that the amygdala, and all the noise it makes, is something inside us, but in no way truly represents us. Mindfulness training teaches that **our authentic inner voice is self-caring and self-protecting,** and that our mission is to find and utilize that voice. Part of the 'dueling' nature is that we have **two competing mental narrators**, telling our stories to ourselves in the world. Our negative narrator announces that we are losers and victims, while our upstairs narrator tells the story of the many obstacles we have overcome and are determined to overcome as we move forward. I recently asked a patient of mine who had a twenty-year history of heroin addiction including seven years in jail, who has now been sober for two years and feeling happier and more stable and better than ever, what helped him to turn things around. He said: "I came in touch with just how much I truly desired a better life for myself!" That is the sound of a true, authentic voice. Desire for a better life arm wrestles and wins the battle with the "craving" for the drug. This in turn, creates more positive and constructive thinking: "I can do it", which must arm wrestle and win the battle with the thought: "I'm incapable." These successful arm-wrestles in turn lead to wiser choices (restraint of self-harming impulsivity) and wiser actions (like choosing to go back to school or get a job).

I also hope you have learned that having negative thoughts, negative feelings, and harmful impulses, does not make you a misfit or alien creature—but rather are the

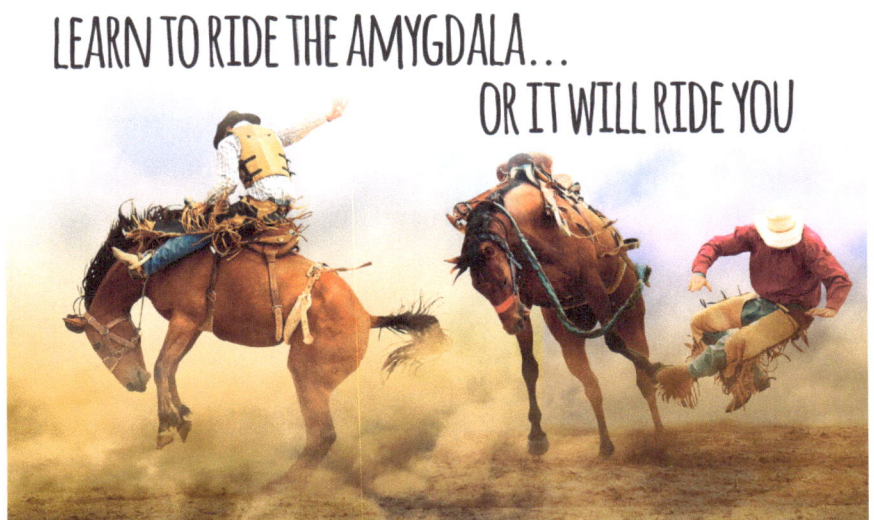

hallmark of your humanity that comes factory-equipped with a remarkable, yet at times troubling, brain. But I also hope you have learned how to at least begin to take the necessary steps to realize the best of your humanity, and now realize you must win the duel with your amygdala to do so.

The amygdala is not bad, and **YOU are not bad because you have one. You are human because you have one.**

But the amygdala is just a **small piece of nerve tissue that served us much better 200,000 years ago then it does now.** We must learn to accept that some parts of our nerve tissues—in fact, most of them—serve us much better than others. The last thing we want to do is identify ourselves with the nerve tissue that does not serve us well—whether that nerve tissue is generating depression, anxiety, or misguided urges to use alcohol or substances. It has some nerve!

If we pause for a moment to assess where we are right now, we might conclude that at this very moment, we are caught between the mistakes we have made in the past, and the mistakes we have yet to make. Conversely, we might also conclude we are caught between the wiser choices we have made in the past, and the wiser choices we have yet to make. I sincerely hope this book has inspired you to make wiser choices as you move forward in your life, and that you feel that reading this book is one of those wiser choices.

If reading this book has been step 1, **what will be your next step?** Re-reading it? Doing the homework? Applying it to your life? Sharing it with a loved one? Changing how you think about the way you think? Cultivating positive thoughts and feelings? Weeding out the negative ones? Holding the door for someone? Catching yourself in the act of overreacting and nipping it in the bud? Putting a mental waste basket in your room?

What inspired me to write this book, was the input and feedback from so many folks to whom I have presented aspects of this novel approach of **understanding ourselves better though understanding our brains better**. The feedback whether it be from individual patients or in rooms filled with hundreds of people has been consistent: "Thank-you, I have never understood myself this well-before!", and "When are you going to write your book?" I hope what is conveyed by such comments and questions is that the people I treat pick up very quickly that I see them more than just as patients, but also as students—and even more so, as fellow human beings. It is in this spirit that I feel it is incumbent upon me **not just to medicate but to educate**.

One of these folks painted the last picture in the book. Her picture of the burdensome suitcases that we all carry and need to let go off to lighten our load showed that she was listening carefully.

Another group member who studied a pre-publication draft of this book and reported that she found the teaching metaphors I used to be quite helpful, went on to write down the metaphors she identified, which became part of the group discussion for the next two weeks, and now are listed in the appendix for all to review. Most who participate in this work develop a "pay it forward" attitude and are eager to share what they have learned with their partners, friends, and family members.

I hope I have lit the fire of your curiosity about yourself, as well as dampened the flame of your judgmentalism and negative self-thinking.

I hope that having read this book, some of your burden has also been lifted, and the path toward further lightening illuminated so that making that effort does not seem so daunting. If you are pressed for time, just read and re-read the Schnappssis I provided at the back of the book, or review the Mindfulness Benefits charts to help you remember and refocus. I wish you and your loved ones the best on your journey to sobriety, well-being, and compassionate self-understanding and change. **The world is awaiting the arrival of your best self. Don't settle for anything less!**

Your feedback is important to me. You can email AckermanPsychiatry@gmail.com and access my website www.AckermanPsychiatry.com

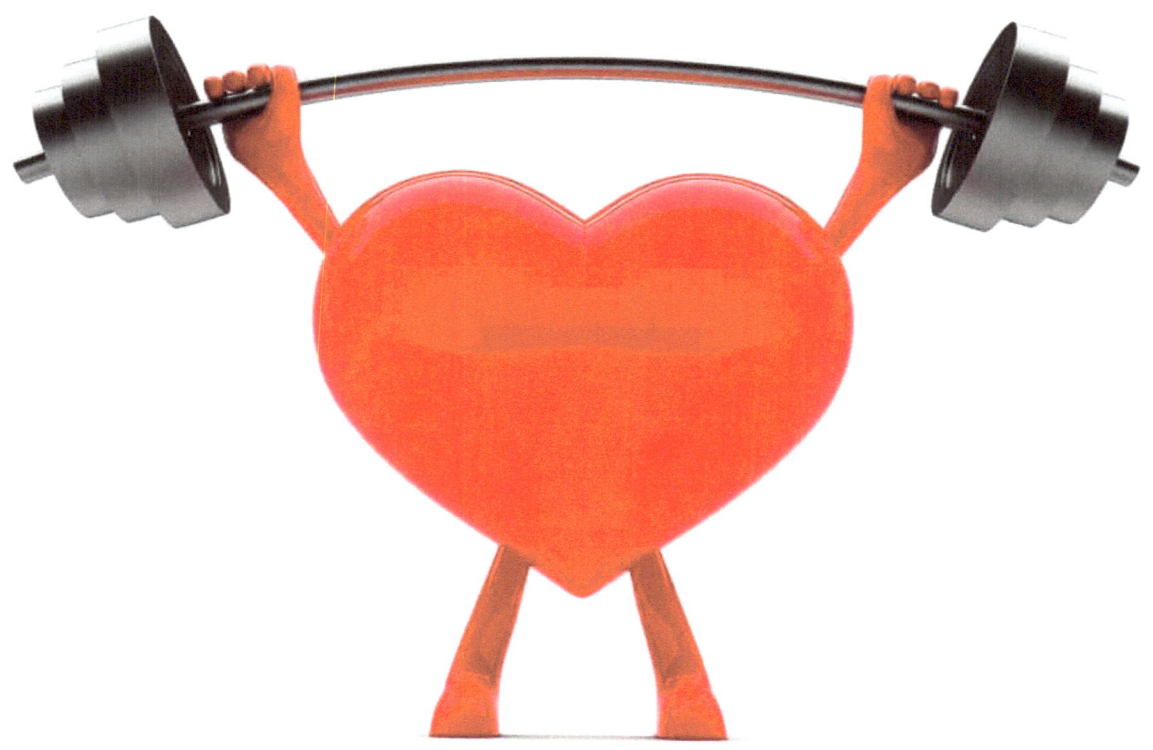

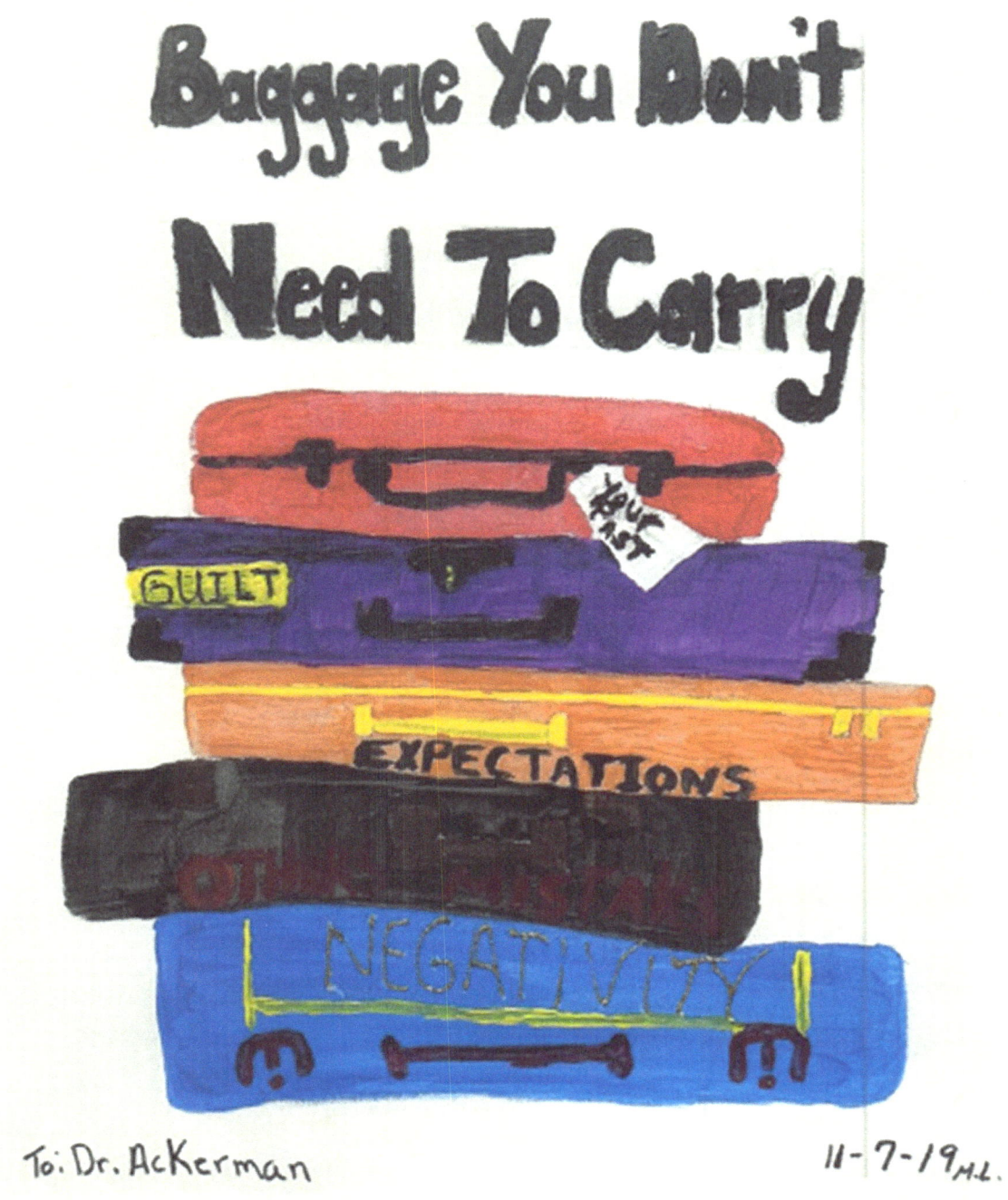

Schnapps-is

Here's what I hope you have learned.

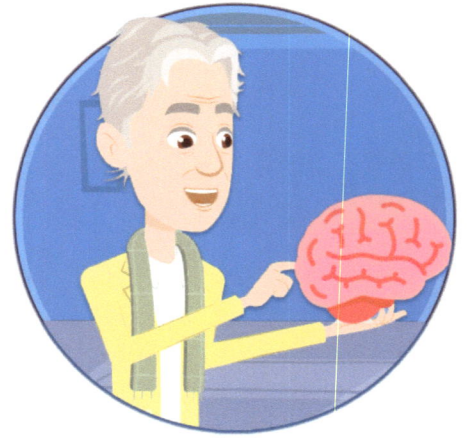

YOU have an amazing human brain!

You have been **UNDERUTILIZING** the **best part of your brain**: your prefrontal cortex. **Your prefrontal cortex is already peaceful.** If you want to feel more peaceful, you have to gain access to and develop this mental room, which is the biggest and best part of your brain. The prefrontal cortex is already peaceful, because it accepts—and does not fight with—reality.

When reality presents some obstacles, the prefrontal cortex immediately welcomes the challenge of problem-solving how to overcome them.

The part of your brain that pushes you to drink, use drugs, or cause harm to yourself or your relationships, friendships, or work life: is YOUR AMYGDALA AND IS REALLY QUITE SMALL. Your amygdala also pushes you to feel lousy, think negative thoughts, and to be impulsive. Your amygdala is your **built-in pusher**. Staying away from the pusher on the streets is one thing; staying away from the pusher in your brain is quite another. Your amygdala is always fighting with reality and so is constantly irritated with all that is. But the amygdala has extremely limited and distorted vision, and does not possess the ability to be aware of its own distortions. When the amygdala comes upon problems, it gets easily irritated. It magnifies their severity and is soon ready to give up in despair about how to overcome them.

YOU are no more a bad person because you have an amygdala any more than you are a bad person if you are nearsighted. Every human being has an amygdala and every human being's life is challenged because of it. Everyone sees themselves with distorted vision.

To get and stay sober, you must take on and win the battle with your amygdala. Drinking and drug use are self-defeating because they make the amygdala stronger. To get well and stay well, you must learn to shrink your amygdala and strengthen your prefrontal cortex.

STOP trying to FIX your brain with drugs. STOP being a SELF-MEDICATOR. Stop trying to be a mechanic to your brain, like you're making adjustments to the engine of your hot rod in your garage. Collaborate with only professionals licensed and experienced in prescribing for alcohol and substance use, to determine what to put into your body that will impact your brain. **The brain is not an organ to tinker with.**

Start taking better care of your brain. Your brain demands that you protect it from harm. You did not read this fine print requirement when you realized you even had a brain, because your brain came with absolutely no care instructions whatsoever. Moreover, impulses to do the opposite: to self-neglect or self-harm are already built-in to your amygdala. Because these self-harming, self-neglecting impulses are built-in, don't locate your problem in the drug, but rather in the part of the brain that, like a pusher, deludes you into thinking just how much you want and "crave" these harmful substances.

In the end, ONLY YOU can decide what to put into your body. 98% of your brain wants nothing to do with drugs or alcohol. The other 2% 'seeks' the "formula" for disaster.

Understanding your brain helps you to understand how and where your wise, intelligent, self-caring, and self-protecting, decisions get made. The secret to this is becoming aware of the small part of your brain that is both impulsive and foolish—to identify it, but not identify with it.

You are capable of making wise, intelligent, self-caring, and self-protecting decisions and can **further help yourself by developing and strengthening** the part of your brain that is designed to do just that.

Mindfulness is a unique feature of our prefrontal cortex which allows us to be aware of possessing this rather amazing brain – and, of its positive and negative features. Once we become aware of its one negative feature, we must learn to not identify ourselves by this feature, but rather to shift our energies into managing this part better, and redirecting our attention to the best part of our brain.

We must learn to become compassionate, non-judgmental witnesses to all our mental noise and to become amused by it, rather than distressed by it.

Your prefrontal cortex is the large, underutilized and underdeveloped room in your brain that houses your best self. It is an incredibly comfortable room, air-conditioned, with comfortable couches and interesting things to do, books to read, music to listen to, and instruments to play. It has an attached screened-in porch that brings you closer to nature and soothing breezes. It is the room where you can pause and think with greater creativity and clarity to better chart your path forward. Guilt, shame, self-recriminations, dwelling on past traumas and past mistakes, are not allowed entry. It is a room where negative thoughts, negative feelings and negative impulses can be nipped in the bud. **Your prefrontal cortex is calling out to you to inhabit this room.** If you become really silent, and listen to its call, you will hear it calling to you imploringly. **You will start feeling better about yourself the moment you step inside**. You will continue to **feel better about yourself** as you learn how to **return to this room every time you need to**—which will be **often.**

Mindfulness training is your treasure map. Follow its directions and it will **take you to your treasure: your best self. When you find it, never let it go.** Learn to treat your best self like one of your children, and nurture your best self to grow and blossom. While there are many who believe that the root of alcohol and substance use problems is the denial and minimization of your substance use, I believe that the even greater root is your denial and minimization of your best self. **Once you let your genie out of your-bottle, you are on the right path.**

The goal of mindfulness training is to **help you discover and release your best self.** When the noted poet Walt Whitman stumbled onto his best self, he described it as follows: "I am larger, better than I thought; I did not know I held so much goodness."

You have held yours back for too long, don't you think?

Schnapps-is

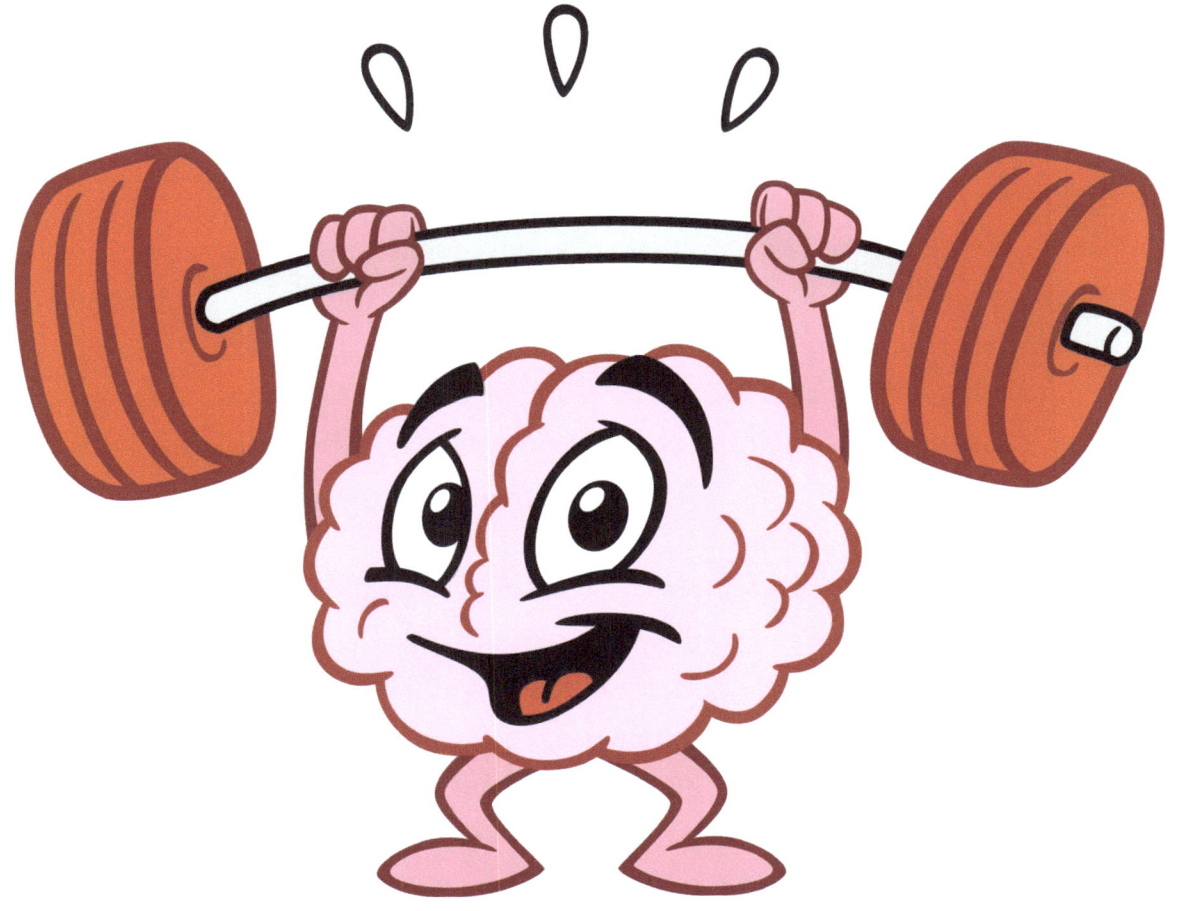

APPENDIX

Reminders

Alcohol and substance use are self-harming & self-defeating behaviors.

Self-defeating behaviors are knee-jerk, automatic, and reflexive in nature and are driven by a small part of the brain that is wired that way. The very best part of your brain is reflective, not reflexive and you can learn, like strengthening your bicep, to develop this part.

Mindfulness training also teaches you consequence awareness and solution awareness.

Thinking you don't care about the consequences is pure nonsense.

Self-defeating behavior is driven by underlying self-contempt and is the culmination of the many ways you have been seeing yourself as weak, defective, a disappointment, a failure. These patterns of negative self-thinking are built into the lower psyche of EVERY human being.

Mindfulness training helps you become aware of the self-defeating impulse, and by learning to "duel" with it successfully, a step at a time, begins the conversion of self-contempt to self-caring determination.

When you learn that your self-contempt comes from your amygdala and how tiny the brain area is, you will get angry for a second, and then become more determined to put this small section of nerve tissue in its proper place. Instead of being your own worst enemy, you can learn to become your own best friend.

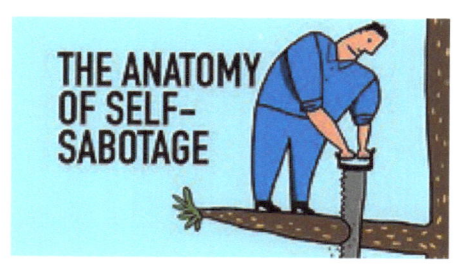

Appendix

Look at the following charts that illustrate, for quick reference reminders: a treasure map of the brain, the physical and mental health benefits of mindfulness practice, and our inherent struggle with our amygdala module. Glance at the charts as often as you can, as they provide helpful reminders. You want these benefits for yourself, no? They are there for you, right at your fingertips. You deserve them. Go get 'em!

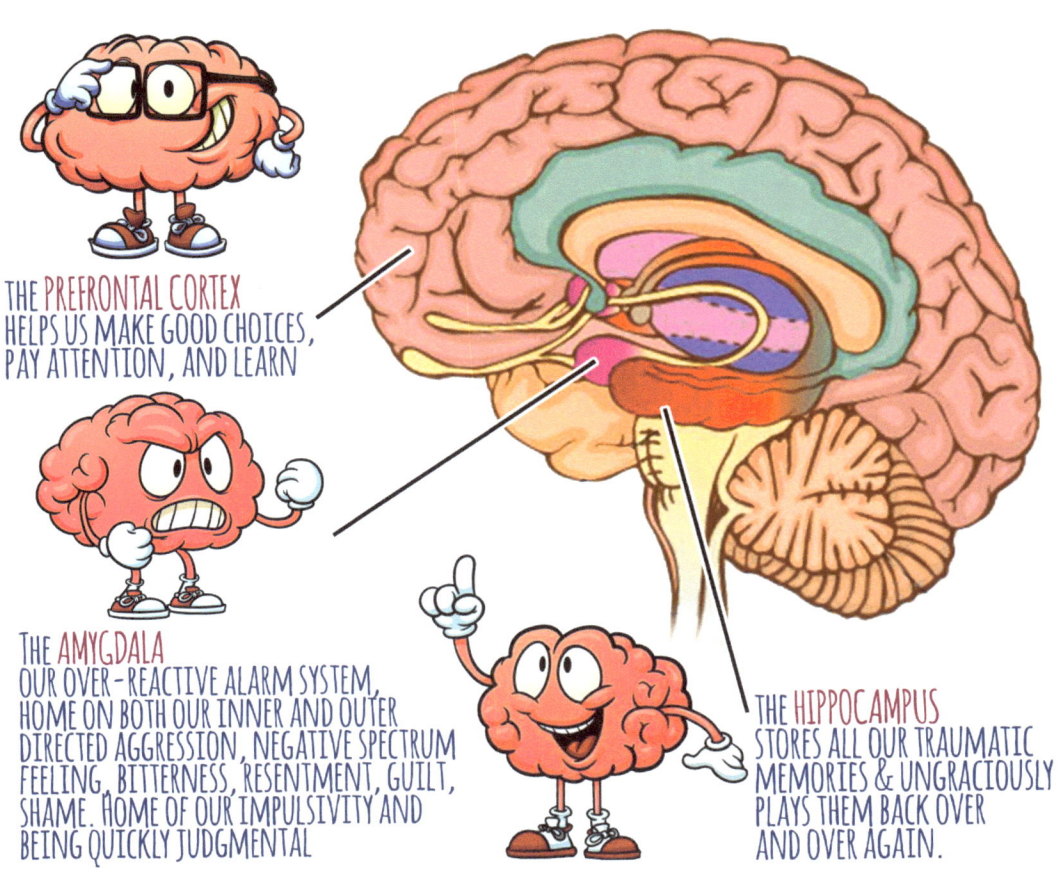

THE PREFRONTAL CORTEX
HELPS US MAKE GOOD CHOICES, PAY ATTENTION, AND LEARN

THE AMYGDALA
OUR OVER-REACTIVE ALARM SYSTEM, HOME ON BOTH OUR INNER AND OUTER DIRECTED AGGRESSION, NEGATIVE SPECTRUM FEELING, BITTERNESS, RESENTMENT, GUILT, SHAME. HOME OF OUR IMPULSIVITY AND BEING QUICKLY JUDGMENTAL

THE HIPPOCAMPUS
STORES ALL OUR TRAUMATIC MEMORIES & UNGRACIOUSLY PLAYS THEM BACK OVER AND OVER AGAIN.

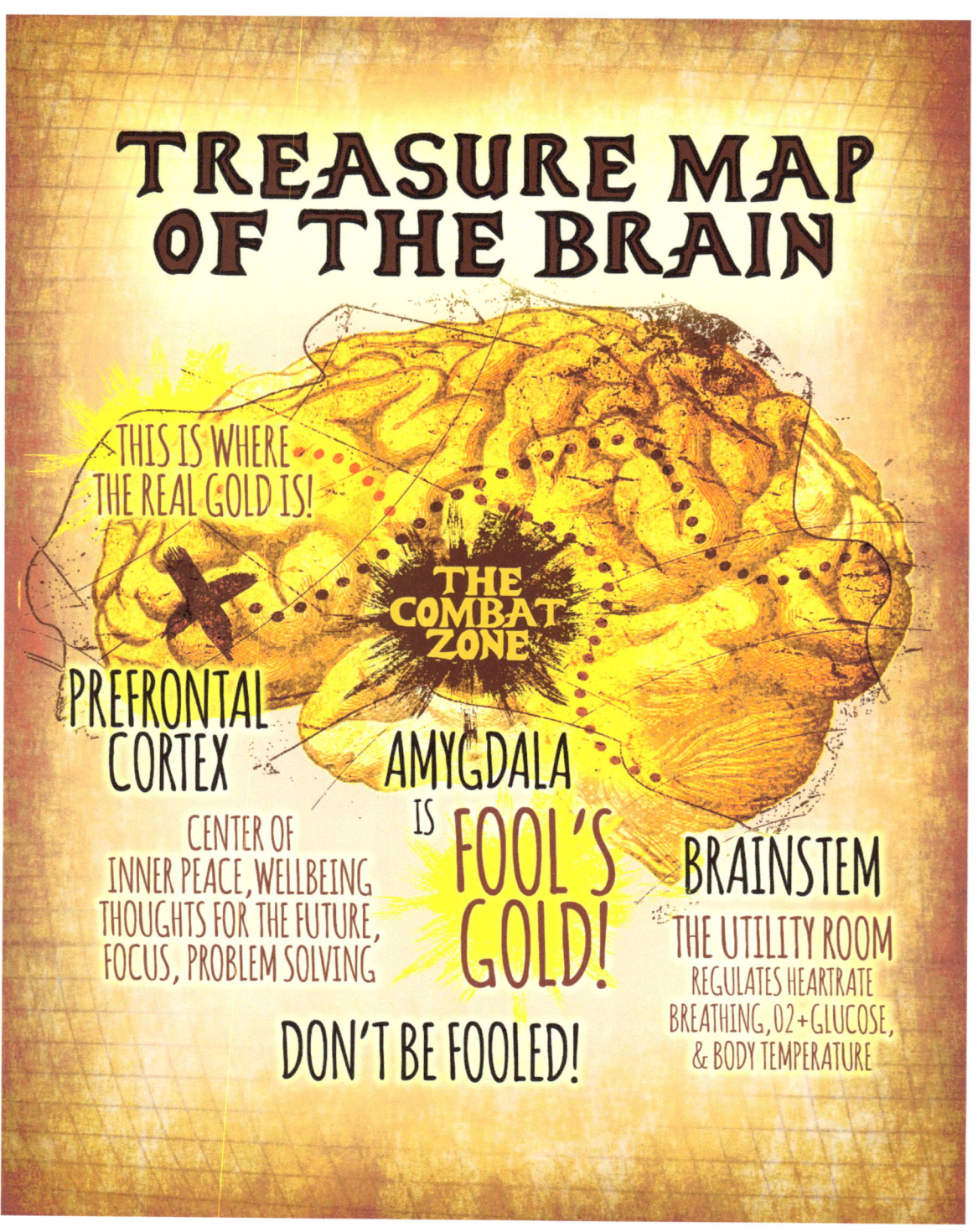

Appendix

AMYGDALA
Your jumpy, irritable, distractible, impulsive, over-reacting drug seeking, wishful thinking lower-psyche, that leads you to react and act without the benefit of the best of our thinking.

HIPPOCAMPUS
Records, stores, and plays back all your negative memories even when they provide no benefit.

Nucleus Accumbens
The pleasure center: filled with Dopamine: **Fools Gold**

TOGETHER THE AMYGDALA, HIPPOCAMPUS & NUCLEUS ACCUMBENS FORM THE **COMBAT ZONE** OF THE BRAIN

Pre-Frontal Cortex
The biggest & best part of your brain that helps you make, good, wise, self and other caring & protecting decisions. **IT CAN LEARN TO OVERRIDE THE COMBAT ZONE.** It keeps its eyes focused on what truly matters, looks to the future and is hopeful. It keeps focused on the pursuit of our inner peace and well-being and is already peaceful because it accepts reality rather than fights with it, and is able and willing to take on and problem-solve all challenges.

Brian L. Ackerman, M.D.

Benefits of Mindfulness

- Sustain Attention and Direct it to what Really Matters
- Helps us Let Go of Feeling like a Victim
- Improve Sense of Well-being
- Become More Joyful and Glad to be Alive
- Helps us Feel More Loving & Compassionate towards Ourselves & Others
- Inspires us to Better Self & Other Care
- Helps us Make Wiser Decisions
- Helps us be Aware of but not Hijacked by our Lower Self
- Helps us Let Go of Resentment & Bitterness
- Cultivate & Nurture our Best Self
- Quiets Negative Thoughts
- Communicate Authentically
- Helps us not Settle for Short-Term Pleasure, but Pursue Long-Term Contentment
- Access Higher, More Creative, Positive Hopeful Thinking
- Helps us Let Go of Shame & Blame
- Helps us Prioritize and Make Better Choices.
- Helps us Nip in the Bud Negative, Self & Other Thinking
- Helps Find more Inner Peace, Joy and Contentment

Teaching Metaphors in Me, Myself & My Amygdala (Prepared for Mindfulness Group by DH)

A. Foreword
   1. Brain owner and operator manual
   2. Snowstorm, snowplow and path to get out

B. What is Mindfulness?
   1. Mental duplex, upstairs apartment and downstairs apartment
   2. Amygdala as an Improvised Explosive Device
   3. Prefrontal cortex as a conductor, brain modules as instruments in an orchestra, amygdala as the drum
   4. Amygdala as a three year old with car keys, prefrontal cortex as parent
   5. The Evolutionary Perspective
   6. Evolution of brain like individual stores in a mall
   7. Best part of brain driver's seat, amygdala distractions that keep us from reaching our destination safely
   8. Brain developed like a rapidly-growing company
   9. Neurons developed like medical specialists
   10. Mindfulness as a person observing on a safari
   11. Unhealthy thoughts as a swamp, healthy thinking as a fresh spring
   12. Amygdala as 911 system and prefrontal cortex as an override
   13. Mental vaccine and mental antibodies for mental anguish
   14. Horrible memories or faulty thinking as an electrical circuit with faulty wiring. Neurons acting as a gas pedal and brake.
   15. Amygdala as the gas pedal, prefrontal cortex the brake.
   16. Mindfulness training as a brake lining to stop negative thinking
   17. Mental lint in the dryer that needs to be cleaned
   18. Mental tennis match between prefrontal cortex and amygdala
   Mental dance between amygdala and prefrontal cortex and mental dance shoes

C. Mental Digestion
   1. Harsh experiences like mental acid reflux
   2. Toxic experiences as mental muck needing excretion as mental waste
   3. Social distancing from mental waste
   4. Mindfulness as a tool selector, negative thoughts loose screws
   5. Amygdala as a built-in negativity generator
   6. Amygdala as a leak on a brain boat
   7. Amygdala as a mental waste maker
        i. As a nest soiler
        ii. Mental polluter
   8. Prefrontal cortex as a sump pump removing water from the amygdala's basement, landscaping to divert the water and prevent the flooding.
   9. Mindfulness as gear shift, amygdala as the sound of grinding gears
   10. Mental windshield, negative thoughts as the film clouding it
   11. Mental toilets to flush away negative thinking
   12. Negative thinking and mental food with no nutritional value
   13. Mental fishermen, throwing back negative feelings and impulses
   14. Judgmentalism as gristle on a steak
   15. Prefrontal cortex as mental homeland security detector

D. The Purpose Driven Mindfulness
   1. Amygdala as rain, mindfulness as the building that protects you from the rain
   2. Prefrontal cortex as air conditioned room, amygdala as a hot room
   3. Amygdala as raining Seattle, prefrontal cortex as Aruba
   4. Higher module the prefrontal cortex, lower module the amygdala
   5. Automobile factory with the amygdala producing the smoke pollution and waste
   6. Brain as a television or radio, mindfulness as the remote choosing best channels
        i. Anxiety channel and depression network
   7. Survival of the mental fittest
   8. Quarantining healthy thoughts from sick thoughts
   9. Harmful thoughts as mental fireflies

Teaching Metaphors in Me, Myself & My Amygdala   (Prepared for Mindfulness Group by DH)

E. The Purpose Driven Mindfulness
  1. Negative co-productions, byproducts and mental waste as unwanted thoughts produced
  2. Non-useful mental productions as exhaust from a car
     i. Smoke from an automobile factory
  3. Mental dialysis as a way to eliminate mental waste
  4. Prefrontal cortex as a Swiss army knife
     i. As a cutting blade

F. Negative Thinking
  1. Prefrontal cortex like a jukebox selecting songs that brings music to the ears
  2. Toxic thoughts held with mental fork in left hand and cut with mental knife (prefrontal cortex) in the right
  3. Separating thoughts like important mail from junk mail thoughts
  4. Separating goods thoughts from bad thoughts like recycling paper, and plastic from trash
  5. Don't let your mind become a dumping ground for noxious experiences like dumping plastics in the ocean
  6. Prefrontal cortex is our driver
     i. Overseer
     ii. Selector in chief
  7. Realizer in chief
  8. Mindfulness homework as mental filtration exercise
  9. Mental oxygen as thoughts feelings and impulses that nourish us
     Quarantine mental carbon dioxide as thought, feelings and impulses that interfere with our well-being

G. Meta-Thinking
  1. Jewelers would carefully examine thoughts like gems accessing quality and usefulness
  2. Fisherman learning to recognize the tugs of love, compassion, kindness, gratitude, and positive thoughts of self-worth and hopefulness on the fishing line
  3. Fisherman releasing tugs of bitterness, resentment, self-hatred, shame and despair
  4. Learning to cool off and ice mental injuries

5. Jeweler not making a quick first glance, but analyzing thoughts with second and third more careful observations
6. Like a baker separating high cholesterol yolks of our lower brain from healthier whites of our upper brain
7. Mental skeet shooting with prefrontal cortex as a rifle shooting down negative thoughts, feelings, and impulses
8. Amygdala like a refrigerator; always running—no off switch

H. The Evolutionary mind(s)
   1. Thoughts like mental fireflies: observe but do not chase and catch
   2. Amygdala as a gas pedal the prefrontal cortex as a brake
   3. The amygdala, nucleus accumbens, and hippocampus (traumatic memory center) like Boston's Combat Zone
   4. Dopamine as Fool's Gold

I. The Role of Trauma
   1. Traumatic memories made with sticky glue, need to let them go
   2. Traumatic memories as bullies to our positive memories

J. Understanding the Prefrontal Cortex
   1. Prefrontal cortex as open for expansion and development
   2. Composting heartache in the soil of future growth
   3. Prefrontal Cortex
      i. as a hand grasping abstract ideas, such as the concepts of illness, well-being, inner peace, awe, love
      ii. as a security guard preventing being hijacked by amygdala
      iii. as a tool with a key to release the handcuffs of the amygdala
      iv. as a CEO of a company making final decisions over other modules middle managing and the amygdala's heckling
      v. as a conductor with other modules playing instruments and the amygdala as a persistent and disruptive drum
      vi. as a loving parent attending the body's nutritional and emotional needs
      vii. as gardener picking fruits and vegetables and picking weeds

Teaching Metaphors in Me, Myself & My Amygdala   (Prepared for Mindfulness Group by DH)

K. Higher Quality versus Lesser Quality Thoughts, Feelings & Impulses
    1. Amygdala as a dog who needs a bone to quiet down

L. Duel Diagnosis
    1. Negative thoughts like bees that sting
        i. Nest in angry, depressed, and anxious thoughts
    2. Stoking the fire of curiosity and dampening the flame of judgmentalism and negative self-thinking

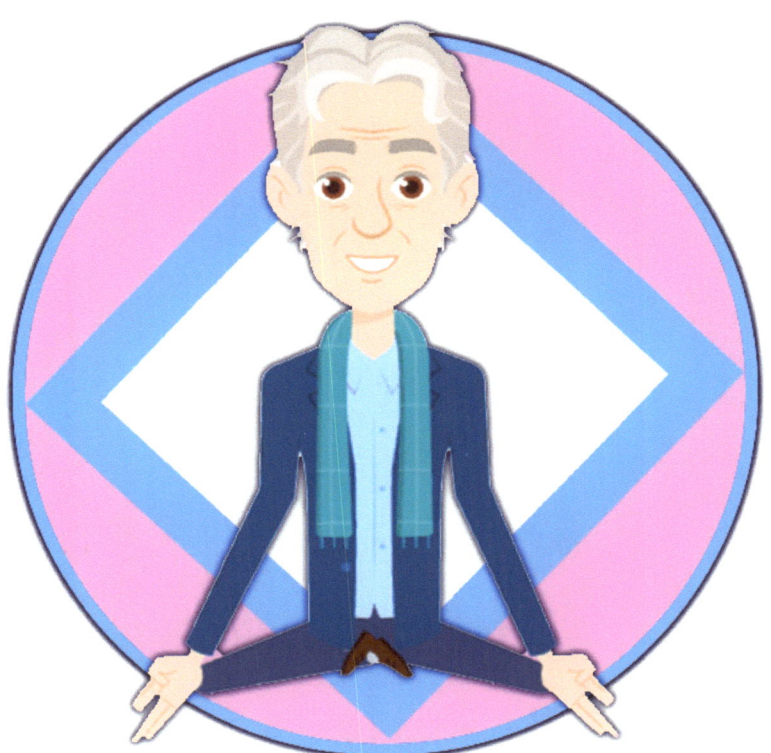

About the Author

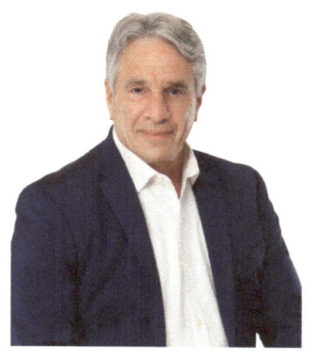
Brian L. Ackerman MD is a Harvard Medical School trained psychiatrist who is the psychiatric medical director of Phoenix House in Rhode Island. He is also the director of Meditation & Mindfulness Services and training at Thrive Behavioral Health, as well as staff psychiatrist at AdCare and Community Care Alliance, where he teaches mindfulness educational groups for staff and patients.

www.ingramcontent.com/pod-product-compliance
Lightning Source LLC
Chambersburg PA
CBHW041504220426
43661CB00016B/1251